Praise for Marion Nestle

"When journalists need to understand how an agricultural policy or nutrition guideline will affect public health, they call Marion Nestle. . . . Nestle has an unparalleled ability to parse USDA reports and cut through the hype to deliver sane, informed nutritional information you can use."—*Time*

"One of the most dogged chroniclers of the U.S. food industry and its politics."—NPR/*The Salt*

"Marion Nestle is a well-respected nutrition expert with degrees in molecular biology and public health nutrition, whose writing is smart and accessible."
—*New York Magazine/The Cut*

"Don't be put off by the fact that she's an academic; Nestle writes in simple and informative language."
—*Vice*

"Nestle has had a hand in changing how food is studied, understood, and even—many would argue—produced."—*Civil Eats*

"[A] longtime crusader on conflicts of interest in food science."—*Vox*

"One of the key voices in food policy, nutrition, and food education in this country."
—*The Village Voice*

"Nestle has made a career of letting people know things the food industry often does its best to obscure. She decodes the gobbledygook on labels and sorts out the good food-health studies from the spin. She documents the many ways the food industry drives government food policy. And she exposes the enormous amounts of money spent to market junk food to kids. . . . Nestle is simply one of the nation's smartest and most influential authorities on nutrition and food policy."
—*San Francisco Chronicle/SF Gate*

"Nestle has been an extraordinary force in shaping the way we think and talk about food."—James Beard Foundation/*Huffington Post*

"Marion Nestle may be America's foremost public nutrition warrior. The scientist, activist, and author has been advocating for clarity in food research and marketing for years, and has been highly critical of the food industry."—*Undark*

Praise for *Food Politics: How the Food Industry Influences Nutrition and Health*

"A courageous and masterful exposé."—Julia Child

"Essential reading for anyone seriously interested in addressing the nutritional dilemma facing the United States."—*Science*

"Provocative and highly readable."—*The Economist*

"An excellent introduction to how decisions are made in Washington—and their effects on consumers." —*The Nation*

"Thought provoking. . . . Voting with our forks for a healthier society, Nestle shows us, is within our power."—*Los Angeles Times*

"Combining the scientific background of a researcher and the skills of a teacher, she has made a complex subject easy to understand. . . . It's hard to argue with Dr. Nestle's point that food is above all political." —*New York Times*

Praise for *Safe Food: The Politics of Food Safety*

"An excellent analysis of the shortcomings of the science-based approach to food."—*The Guardian*

"Provocative and consumer-friendly."—*Saveur*

"Nestle lets us in on conversations we'd never otherwise hear. What we learn may be more than we can stomach. . . . *Safe Food* weighs in on all the hot topics."—*San Francisco Chronicle*

"Marion Nestle speaks in a voice that is by turns that of a consumer advocate and a scientist." —*The Boston Globe*

Also written or edited by Marion Nestle

Nutrition in Clinical Practice (1985)

The Surgeon General's Report on Nutrition and Health (edited with J. Michael McGinnis, 1988)

Food Politics: How the Food Industry Influences Nutrition and Health (2002; revised edition 2007; tenth anniversary edition 2013)

Safe Food: The Politics of Food Safety (2003; revised edition 2010)

Taking Sides: Clashing Views on Controversial Issues in Nutrition and Food (edited with L. Beth Dixon, 2004)

What to Eat (2006)

Pet Food Politics: The Chihuahua in the Coal Mine (2008)

Feed Your Pet Right (with Malden C. Nesheim, 2010)

Why Calories Count: From Science to Politics (with Malden C. Nesheim, 2012)

Eat, Drink, Vote: An Illustrated Guide to Food Politics (2013)

Soda Politics: Taking on Big Soda (and Winning) (2015)

Big Food: Critical Perspectives on the Global Growth of the Food and Beverage Industry (edited with Simon N. Williams, 2016)

Unsavory Truth: How Food Companies Skew the Science of What We Eat (2018)

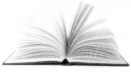

The publisher and the University of California Press Foundation gratefully acknowledge the generous support of the Simpson Imprint in Humanities.

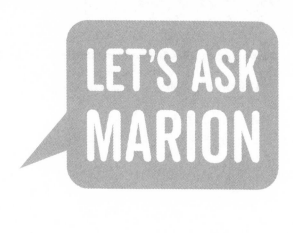

California Studies in Food and Culture

Darra Goldstein, Editor

LET'S ASK MARION

WHAT YOU NEED TO KNOW ABOUT THE POLITICS OF FOOD, NUTRITION, AND HEALTH

MARION NESTLE

in conversation with

Kerry Trueman

UNIVERSITY OF CALIFORNIA PRESS

University of California Press
Oakland, California

© 2020 by Marion Nestle and Kerry Trueman

Cataloging-in-Publication Data is on file at
    the Library of Congress.
ISBN 978-0-520-34323-8 (cloth : alk. paper)
ISBN 978-0-520-97469-2 (ebook)

Design and composition: Lia Tjandra
Printing: Versa Press

Manufactured in the United States of America

28 27 26 25 24 23 22 21 20
10 9 8 7 6 5 4 3 2 1

CONTENTS

II. THE COMMUNITY POLITICS OF FOOD CHOICE

III. THE GLOBAL POLITICS OF DIETS, HEALTH, AND THE ENVIRONMENT

INTRODUCTION

When my book *Food Politics* first appeared in 2002, the immediate reaction to its title was "What does politics have to do with food?" Years later, I am still asked that question. This book aims to answer it. To begin with, the food we consume and enjoy every day is influenced, if not determined, by the power of food companies to sell products, no matter how those products might affect our health or that of our planet. We are obliged to eat in order to obtain the nutrients and energy we need to grow, reproduce, and survive. Here, I describe why and how a substance essential for our very existence has become a touchstone for political disputes about culture, identity, social class, inequity, and power, as well as arguments about what roles are appropriate for government, private enterprise, and civil society in twenty-first-century democratic societies.

Although trained in basic science (my Berkeley doctorate was in molecular biology), I have spent most of my professional career as a public health nutritionist and food studies academic. From this perspective, today's greatest public health nutrition problems—the Big Three—are hunger (affecting roughly a billion people globally), obesity (two billion and rising), and climate change (everybody). These share at least one cause in common: all are due in part to dysfunctional food systems, a term that encompasses everything that happens to a food from production to consumption. Food systems, in turn, depend on political and economic systems. If we want to eliminate hunger, prevent the health consequences of excessive weight gain, and protect the environment, we must understand, confront, and counter the political forces that created these problems and allow them to continue.

For decades, I have been thinking, writing, publishing, and teaching about how politics affects and distorts food systems. If anything has changed over these years, it is the explosion of public interest in the politics of food, and in advocating for food systems that better support health and the environment. The goal of much of my recent work has been to inspire not only "voting with forks" for healthier and more environmentally sustainable personal diets, but also "voting with votes." By this I mean engaging in politics to advocate for food systems that make better food available and affordable to everyone, that adequately compensate everyone who works to produce, prepare, or serve food, and that deal with food in ways that conserve and sustain the environment.

Since 2002, I have written, edited, co-authored, or co-edited the books about the politics of food listed at the front of this book. These include hundreds of pages of detailed discussion, exhaustively referenced. Despite my best efforts to make my writing clear and accessible, my books must seem daunting, because I am often asked for a shorter summary of their principal points. I have resisted, not only because I want people to read my books, but also because I do not find short essays easy to write. From 2008 to 2013, I wrote a monthly column for the food section of the *San Francisco Chronicle.* These columns were supposed to respond to readers' questions, but few readers asked any, which made writing them hard work.

In contrast, I very much enjoyed responding to questions from my friend Kerry Trueman, a dedicated environmental advocate who frequently blogged about food issues and occasionally asked my opinion about whatever she was writing about. At some point, she began asking more formal questions and posting our exchanges under the heading "Let's Ask Marion." I co-posted these exchanges on the blog I have written since 2007 at www.foodpolitics.com.

Kerry's questions were sometimes about specific events in the news, sometimes about more general topics. What she asked reflected her highly informed concerns about the intersection of dietary choices and agricultural practices, and I appreciated her intuitive food-systems thinking. Her questions ranged from the personal to the political, from food production to consumption, and from the domestic to the international. They often challenged me to think about issues I might not otherwise have considered and were so much fun to deal with that I could quickly respond. In searching for a relatively uncomplicated way to write short accounts of my current thinking about food-system issues, I wondered whether Kerry would consider working with me to produce a book in a question-and-answer format. Happily, she agreed. This book is the result of our joint efforts and would not have been possible without her collaboration.

My overarching purpose in writing these short essays is to encourage advocacy for food systems that are healthier for people and the planet. Successful advocacy means engaging in politics to counter the actions of a food industry narrowly focused on profit, all too often at the expense of public health. In this book, I use "food industry" to refer to the companies that produce, prepare, serve, and sell food, beverages, and food products. Although this industry includes agricultural producers and restaurant companies, most of my discussion is about the companies that raise or make the foods and food products that we typically buy in supermarkets.

In the current political era, the methods used by the food industry to sell products, regardless of health consequences, are largely unchecked by government regulation. This is because the governments of many countries, including our own, have been strongly influenced—"captured"—by industry. Also, in many countries, civil society is too weak to effectively demand curbs on industry marketing practices. Advocacy means organizing civil society and pressing government to create healthier and more sustainable food systems. This means politics.

In trying to decide what this book should cover, Kerry and I thought the questions should address how politics affects personal dietary choices, the food environment in communities (in the United States and elsewhere), and the truly global nature of current food systems, and we organized the questions under those three categories. Within each category, we wanted to include the questions we hear most frequently, along with those that illustrate why and how food is political and what needs to be done to make foods systems better for everyone, poor as well as rich. Across the categories and questions, several themes come up repeatedly. Watch for these themes in particular.

Food is one of life's greatest pleasures. I list this first because it underlies all of my thinking about food and food issues. Food is delicious as well as nourishing and is one of the supreme joys of human culture.

Food is political. Because everyone eats, everyone has a stake in the food system, but the principal stakeholders—food producers, manufacturers, sellers, farm and restaurant workers, eaters—do not have the same agenda or power. We eaters want food to be available, affordable, culturally appropriate, healthy, and delicious; workers want to make a decent living; producers and other industry stakeholders want to make a profit. Such interests can and do conflict, especially when profits take precedence over social values of health, equity, and environmental protection.

"Food system" helps explain food issues. As noted earlier, this term refers to the totality of how a food is grown or raised, stored, transported, processed, prepared, sold, and consumed or wasted. Knowing how foods are produced explains much about their availability, cost, and health and environmental consequences. Food systems operate in the context of broader social, cultural, and economic systems; these too have political dimensions.

"Ultraprocessed" is a more precise term for "junk" foods. It refers specifically to products that are industrially produced, bear no resemblance to the foods from which they were extracted, and contain additives never found in home kitchens. Research increasingly links consumption of ultraprocessed foods to poor health.

The principles of healthful diets are well established. We can argue about the details, but diets that promote human health are largely (but not necessarily exclusively) plant-based, provide adequate but not excessive calories, and minimize or avoid ultraprocessed foods. Such diets are also better for the environment.

The food industry influences food choices. Cultural, social, and economic factors influence food choices, but so do food industry marketing and lobbying actions. The food industry's primary job is to sell products and return profits to stockholders; health and environmental considerations are decidedly secondary, if not irrelevant.

Food systems affect the environment. A sustainable (or, in current terms, agroecological or regenerative) food system replaces the nutrients extracted from soil by food plants, and minimizes the damaging effects of animal and plant production on soil, water, and greenhouse gases.

Food systems generate and perpetuate inequities. An ideal food system makes healthy, sustainable, affordable, and culturally appropriate food available and affordable to everyone and enables everyone to have the power to choose such foods, regardless of income, class, race, gender, or age. It adequately compensates workers employed on farms and in meat-packing plants, food production facilities, and restaurants. The goals of food system advocacy are to achieve these ideals.

Kerry and I finished writing this book before the coronavirus-induced respiratory disease, Covid-19, devastated lives, livelihoods, and economies. In exposing the contradictions and inequities of profit-driven economic, health care, and food systems, this global pandemic illustrated our book's themes. In the United States, Covid-19 proved most lethal to the poor, racial minorities, the elderly, and those with obesity-associated chronic diseases. Suddenly, low-wage slaughterhouse and grocery store workers—often migrants or immigrants, and many without sick leave or health care benefits—were deemed *essential*. Slaughterhouses, now viral epicenters, were forced to remain open. Farmers destroyed unsold animals and produce while the newly unemployed lined up at food banks. Corporations laid off workers but took millions in government bailouts and paid salaries and bonuses to executives. These events call for advocacy for strong democratic government and institutions, among them food systems that benefit all members of society, regardless of income, class, citizenship, race, ethnicity, gender, or age.

A Word about the Sources and Further Reading

Because my writings deal with controversial topics—alas, not everyone agrees with my views—I usually make sure to back up nearly every statement with extensive references. But for this book, which draws on so much of my own work, I instead include chapter-by-chapter lists of relevant books, reports, and articles, followed by a list of additional books and reports that have informed my work, some historical, some current. All of these references are meant as starting points for deeper investigation of the issues discussed here.

My hope is that this book succeeds in providing a brief overview of my thinking about food system issues, from the personal to the global. Even more, I hope that it inspires readers to take food politics seriously and to engage in advocacy for healthier, more sustainable, and more equitable food systems for current and future generations.

I

THE POLITICS OF PERSONAL DIETS AND HEALTH

1 WHAT IS A HEALTHY DIET?

Kerry: Marion, do you ever have any nostalgia for the era when whole-grain crackers tasted like dog biscuits and the term "health food" actually scared a lot of people? I'm thinking of the 1960s, when health food stores started to proliferate and earned a reputation for selling obscure foodstuffs that sounded weird and tasted worse.

Now that eating healthfully has become a much more mainstream goal, marketing mavens eager to exploit that admirable aspiration bestow a "health halo" on everything from almond milk to zucchini "zoodles." I'm delighted that consumer demand has encouraged conventional supermarket chains to expand their fresh produce departments, and that quick-serve restaurants are doing well by offering healthier alternatives.

But sadly, this genuine desire to embrace healthier

eating habits also makes consumers more vulnerable to cynical marketing ploys. How do you cut through the marketing hype to give people simple, solid dietary guidelines for eating healthfully?

Marion: Not as easily as I would like. One of the great achievements of today's intense interest in food—a food movement on its own—is the increased availability and variety of fresh fruits and vegetables in most supermarkets in the United States. For those of us who can afford to buy whatever foods we want, eating healthfully and deliciously should be easy. Not so, apparently. That people are confused about food choices is a given. That's why I wrote *What to Eat* in 2006, taking 500 pages to explain how to make sensible choices in every section of a supermarket. In 2015, the U.S. government's "Dietary Guidelines for Americans" used 150 pages to offer its recommendations, and in 2019 an international commission took 50 pages to propose dietary principles for planetary health. The great irony is that basic dietary principles are so easy to explain that the journalist Michael Pollan could summarize them in just seven words: "Eat food. Not too much. Mostly plants."

Really, that's all there is to it. But if following this advice seems impossibly complicated, it's surely because of everything else we are supposed to do when we decide what to eat: meet needs for required nutrients; promote our health and longevity; prevent obesity and the risks it poses for type 2 diabetes, heart disease, and other such conditions; and, in this era of global warming, minimize environmental damage. Foods also have to be affordable, accessible, appropriate to our cultural heritage and preferences, and, of course, taste good. Achieving all this is a tall order for anyone.

Even more, we are expected to make wise choices in the midst of an industry-driven food environment explicitly created to encourage us to eat more of the most profitable food products, anywhere, any time of day or night, and in large amounts. Dealing with today's high-pressure food environment is the principal challenge faced by any health-conscious eater.

Coping with pressures to eat more is an evolutionary challenge. We must eat to live, and we evolved as omnivores. Our Paleolithic hunter-gatherer ancestors ate anything they could get their hands on, learning the hard way to avoid poisonous plants and rotten meat. We exist today only because those ancestors figured out how to hunt and gather sufficient food safely enough to reach reproductive age.

As they also figured out how to cultivate plants, tame animals, and invent agriculture, ancestral humans still struggled to get enough to eat. Even so, they were able to create meals from whatever foods they had available, eventually turning them into cuisines of astonishing variety and deliciousness. The traditional diets of many populations—those in Japan and the Mediterranean, for example—especially promoted health and longevity. Another irony: appreciation for the taste and value of such diets has now put their price beyond the reach of many people in the societies that invented them.

Traditional diets met Pollan's three conditions. Let's start with "eat food." Hunting meant chasing animals; gathering meant collecting edible plants. We did not evolve to eat what Pollan calls "food-like objects," products in packages, with long lists of ingredients, made to last for years—what I call "junk" foods and what Carlos Monteiro, the Brazilian professor of nutrition and public health, more politely calls "ultraprocessed."

Unless picked straight off a tree or vine, any food we buy has been processed to some extent, even if it has only been washed or chopped. But "ultraprocessed" specifically refers to industrially manufactured food products loaded with added sugars, fats, and salt and constructed from ingredients we can't easily make at home, such as artificial flavors, colors, and texturizers. Consider, for example, ways to eat corn: on the cob (unprocessed), canned (processed), Dorito Nacho Cheese Tortilla Chips (ultraprocessed).

By distinguishing ultraprocessed from less extreme forms of processing, Monteiro hit on something quite profound. The distinction enables scientists to compare the effects of eating ultraprocessed to less-processed foods. Such studies are pouring in. They clearly link diets based largely on ultraprocessed food products to increased risks for obesity, type 2 diabetes, heart disease, and overall mortality.

We eat highly processed foods because we love their taste and crunch. Of course we do, and so do our kids. Food companies spend fortunes researching how to appeal to our tastes and to convince us to buy their products. As a result of government policies aimed at keeping the price of junk-food ingredients low, ultraprocessed foods are relatively inexpensive. To pick just two examples: Federal subsidies of corn and soybeans, key ingredients in many ultraprocessed foods, encourage farmers to overproduce these crops, thereby increasing supply relative to demand. And tax laws permit food companies to deduct advertising costs as business expenses, which means that taxpayers effectively subsidize the cost of marketing ultraprocessed foods to children.

One other point: since 1980 or so, the cost of all U.S. foods has increased but the cost of fruits and vegetables has gone up much higher than average. In contrast, the cost of ultraprocessed foods has risen more slowly, making these foods relatively cheap. That is one reason why America's food habits seem class-based. Wealthier and better educated people are more likely to eat healthfully and avoid ultraprocessed foods. Those without such resources do the best they can but may well have to choose diets on the basis of price and convenience rather than health. It doesn't help that billions of dollars of food marketing specifically targets low-income and minority groups. It's easy for me to say "avoid ultraprocessed foods," but not everyone has the means, the ability, or the time to follow that advice.

"Mostly plants" is also easier said than done. If you don't have much money, fruits and vegetables can seem not worth the trouble. They don't feel as filling, spoil easily, take time to prepare, appear expensive, and *are* expensive. Ultraprocessed products are backed by enormous advertising budgets; fruits and vegetables are not.

I view "not too much" as a call for government to take responsibility for creating a healthier food environment. We can vote with our forks—take personal responsibility—for our food choices, but doing so in the face of food-industry pressures to eat more of highly profitable ultraprocessed products is hard to do on our own. We need help. We would have a much easier time following dietary advice in a more health-focused food environment.

I can think of plenty of ways to create one, starting with reducing the cost of basic foods, ending subsidies for ultraprocessed foods, and putting some curbs on food-industry marketing practices, especially those aimed at children. For that we need to vote with our vote—engage in politics and advocate. How to do that deserves its own discussion, which I will get to in the concluding chapter.

2 WHY DOES NUTRITION ADVICE ALWAYS SEEM TO BE CHANGING?

Kerry: Why are so many Americans deeply skeptical—or even downright hostile—toward nutrition science, while millions of us eagerly embrace all kinds of dubious dietary advice dished up by slender celebrities with even more slender credentials?

I blame this schizophrenic attitude in part on decades of self-serving food industry–funded studies that can read like propaganda. But even legitimate research conducted by scientists with sterling credentials sometimes yields confusing results and conflicting answers.

Take the eternal debates over the benefits of products like coffee, wine, or eggs. Are these foods good for us or not? We all want certainty and simplicity, but the science seems to keep changing, so we get frustrated and shrug it all off. How to explain this cognitive dissonance?

Marion: I make no claim to being a psychologist, but it seems to me your question comes down to one of trust. Food is intimate; we put it inside our bodies. But then what happens? Except for what we excrete, we can't see how food is metabolized and used. We can only interpret. Everyone eats. Everyone can claim first-hand experience and expertise.

Whose experience and expertise should you trust? "Mine, of course," is my standard (slightly facetious) answer. I can understand why people trust celebrities more than scientists or nutritionists; they feel like friends, even if the relationship is unreal. It doesn't help that nutritionists have impenetrably confusing credentials, ranging from none beyond personal experience to years of graduate and post-graduate study. I call myself a nutritionist, and hold New York State Nutrition and Dietetics license number 000007 on the basis of a doctoral degree in molecular biology, a master's degree in public health nutrition, and membership on the committee that established that license.

It also doesn't help that nutrition science is so extraordinarily difficult to do. Just think of what it would take to show whether eggs, the largest dietary source of cholesterol, raise the risk of heart disease. To achieve definitive results, you would need to put large numbers of people matched in age, gender, and risk on one of two defined diets, the same except for whether eggs are included. To make sure your study subjects stick to the diet, you would have to confine them under close supervision for expensively long periods to see whether eggs induced symptoms. Humans are not lab rats. We make terrible experimental animals. This forces nutrition scientists to resort to indirect measures, such as blood cholesterol levels, that do not always relate clearly to disease risk.

I've long said that the most intellectually challenging problem in nutrition is to figure out what people eat. Diets vary from day to day, and yours differs from mine. Scientists ask us to write down everything we ate yesterday (twenty-four-hour recall), or to keep track of what we eat in a day (twenty-four-hour dietary record), or to fill out a survey of how often we ate a given food in the last week, month, or year (food-frequency questionnaire). The accuracy of these methods depends on how well we remember what we ate. They are, to say the least, imprecise. At the moment, better methods are too expensive and difficult to use with large numbers of people, leaving researchers to do the best they can with whatever information they can get.

Linking dietary intake to disease risk is also difficult. Suppose you want to know whether people who eat eggs have higher levels of cholesterol in their blood. Food cholesterol raises blood cholesterol, but saturated fat raises it even more. If your blood cholesterol is high, it's hard to know whether this is due to eggs, your level of physical activity, or something else you ate, took, did, or were born with.

That is why the best that most studies can do is to show some kind of association or link between what you ate and the likelihood—your risk—of developing a disease. They cannot prove that what you ate caused a disease. Depending on how studies of eggs and health are designed, the results could go one way or the other— and they do, with no resolution in sight.

A further complication is that the egg industry pays for research about eggs and health. When scientists first identified cholesterol as a risk factor for heart disease, they advised limiting egg intake to no more than one a day. Alarmed, the egg industry commissioned research to cast doubt on that advice. As with much industry-funded research, the egg industry's studies showed "funding effects"—results that favor the sponsor's interests—in this case, that eggs pose no risk to health. Egg research results are now so muddled that the 2015 Dietary Guidelines for Americans judged a limit on dietary cholesterol as unnecessary but advised eating as little cholesterol (meaning as few eggs) as possible. I have no idea what to make of this.

It's not that all industry-funded research is biased; it's just that most of it appears to be. Because nutrition research is so complicated—and because everyone feels like an expert—biases get into this research in all sorts of ways. My molecular biology training has proved useful for dealing with them. As a graduate student, I was taught to distrust my own results and to overcompensate for biases, recognized and not. Scientists are people too. We have hypotheses we want to prove. Some of us may be so wedded to hypotheses that we discount studies we don't like and "cherry-pick" the data. But rigorously trained scientists go out of our way to control for our conscious and unconscious biases.

As it happens, I just love the complexities of nutrition research and findings that are gray, rather than black or white, and that inevitably require interpretation. It is human nature to think that other people are biased, but never ourselves. It is human nature to trust the nutrition opinions of celebrities, even if a moment's thought ought to reveal the absurdity of that trust. A mere trace of critical thinking should make you surprised (if not outraged) that celebrities who know nothing of the complexities of nutrition science are taken seriously as diet gurus, that food companies pay for studies that give them the results they want, and that scientists wedded to their own hypotheses insist that only one diet—the one they recommend—is appropriate for health.

Any nutritionist who thinks critically knows that diets of enormous variety are capable of supporting health and longevity. Except for avoiding food allergies, a claim that one diet, one food, one food product, or one supplement is the solution to your health problems—no matter who that advice comes from—requires skepticism. Critical thinking is especially in order whenever a recommended diet:

involves a product: Here, the claims are likely to be about marketing, not science. Food companies fund research because it helps them sell products. Beware of anyone hawking products of one kind or another.

excludes whole categories of foods: This may help reduce calorie intake but limits variety and pleasure and could lead to reduced intake of certain nutrients. Animal food products are the main source of vitamin B_{12}, for example.

is announced with absolute certainty: That's not how science works. Nutrition science is inherently uncertain due to the complexity of everything we eat, drink, or do.

claims to prevent a wide range of conditions: I get suspicious whenever I see a claim that one food or product will not only prevent type 2 diabetes and heart disease, but also conditions without known cures, such as autism, Alzheimer's, or other cognitive problems.

is advertised as a breakthrough: This too is not how science works. Nutrition science builds on previous studies and makes incremental progress.

insists that everything you thought you knew about nutrition is wrong: Science rarely works this way, so it's best to read the fine print. Case in point: even when health authorities advised cutting down on eggs, they said one a day was acceptable. They still give the same advice.

These same principles apply to studies of coffee, wine, and any other food or drink. As is ever true, the basic principles of nutrition are easily summarized:

Eat a wide variety of foods. Because food plants and animals differ in nutrient composition, variety ensures the full complement of needed nutrients.

Eat relatively unprocessed foods. These contain nutrients but do not have excessive amounts of added sugars, fats, salt, and calories.

Eat in moderation. The word "moderation" may sound like a nutritional joke—what does it mean, exactly?—but the advice aims to keep calorie intake balanced with calorie needs.

To these principles, I would add one more: **Enjoy what you eat.**

How does politics affect these principles? Think about today's "eat more" food environment and what would happen to the food industry if we all ate this way.

3 ARE LOW-CARB DIETS REALLY BETTER FOR US?

Kerry: Passing judgment on other people's dietary choices when they haven't asked for my two cents is just wrong. But I cringe a little when my anti-carb friends insist that a grain-free/gluten-free/high-fat/Paleo/Keto diet can banish belly fat, cure brain fog, and prevent every disease you can name and then some.

I can sympathize, because like a hundred million other Americans, according to the CDC, I have dangerously high blood sugar. It was a sad day when I learned that our bodies convert bagels to sugar in, well, a New York minute.

Overconsumption of sugary drinks, white bread, pizza, and pasta is certainly rampant in our culture, so there's a grain of truth fueling the carbophobia. But tarring *all* carbs with the same pastry brush, or giving the high five to wildly high-fat diets, sounds awfully unbalanced to me. Then again, what if the low-carb zealots are right?

Marion: Ah yes, dietary zealotry. Here's my promise: I won't say a word about what you are eating if you promise never to say to me, "You eat *that*?" Yes, I do. I'm an omnivore. My diet most definitely includes carbohydrates: simple (sugars) and complex (starches), whole (unprocessed) and refined (processed). I'm not sure I've ever met a carb I didn't like.

I say this with some trepidation because whenever I publicly confess my fondness for all things carbohydrate, I am besieged by passionate adherents to low-carb/high-fat diets who are appalled that I do not agree that sugars are poison (they induce insulin), starches are poison (they're converted to sugars), and cutting carbs is the best—if not the only—way to stave off whatever ails you. If I'm not anti-sugar, they insist, I must be part of the scientific conspiracy that for decades has foisted low-fat diets upon us.

No on all counts. Carbs are not poison. We *need* them, for energy and fuel for our brains. I'm guessing that one reason why the arguments about carbs versus fats are so intense is the complexity of their chemistry and metabolism. Small amounts of different kinds of sugars occur naturally in otherwise nutritious fruits, dairy products, and an occasional vegetable. Sugars are more concentrated in honey and maple syrup, but hardly anyone eats much of those.

That is why the only sugars that concern nutritionists like me are the ones extracted from cane, beets, and corn—those listed on food labels as "added sugars." These come with no nutrients (hence empty calories). Most of us eat and drink way too much of them and would be healthier consuming less. But less does not necessarily mean none. Current advice is to keep sugar intake to a limit of 10 percent of daily calories, which for most people comes to about 50 grams, or 12 teaspoons. This is not exactly abstemious.

The main sources of complex carbohydrates are starchy grains—wheat, rice, corn. These, let's remember, have fueled entire civilizations. Even in the modern era, populations with the greatest longevity have been Mediterraneans, who include bread or pasta at practically every meal, and rice-eating Asians.

Fat isn't poison either. Forgive my getting didactic, but we require fat for its content of the omega-3s and omega-6s you hear so much about. Fats of any kind are highest in calories—9 per gram, as opposed to 4 each for carbohydrates or protein—which is why fats are fattening. Saturated fatty acids raise blood cholesterol levels. Animal fats are more saturated than vegetable fats—yet another reason why vegetables are healthier.

But I have a hard time thinking about either fats or carbs outside of their dietary context. Hardly anyone eats sugar, butter, or vegetable oil straight. The real concern should be the foods they come with, how processed those foods are, and how many calories they provide. Relatively unprocessed foods contain vitamins and minerals along with their carbohydrates and fats. Food plants provide fiber, which feeds the bacteria in our intestines—our newly measurable and therefore fascinating microbiome.

Of course exceptions exist. Hard candy and soft drinks provide calories but nothing else of nutritional value, and sweetened beverages account for nearly half the sugars consumed by Americans. The next biggest source is what the USDA charmingly calls "grain-based desserts"—donuts, pies, cakes, cookies, and the like; these are also high in complex carbs. So are bread, pizza, and pasta, but these are usually eaten with butter, oils, or cheese that slow down carbohydrate absorption.

Fruit juices are one more exception. They are processed, but not highly. If you eat one orange or apple, it's usually enough. Hardly anyone would eat four at a time, yet a glass of juice can easily be extracted from that many and have as much sugar as a soft drink. When I was a child, juice glasses held four ounces. That's still a good idea.

Low-carb dieters say they feel better and maintain healthier weights when they avoid those foods. Of course they do; they are consuming fewer calories, losing weight, and reducing disease risks, at least if they avoid overcompensating with calories from fatty foods. It's hard to argue with results like these, and I won't.

As for type 2 diabetes, its most important risk factor is being overweight. This is a calorie problem, not necessarily a carbohydrate problem. Low-fat diets work just as well for weight loss, although they may be harder to stick with; fatty foods taste good and satisfy.

Some people may manage calories better on high-fat diets, but not me, and I find foods with *both* carbs and fats even harder to resist. I can't eat just one French fry, and let's not even talk about ice cream.

We are born loving the taste of sugars in breast milk, and we quickly learn to love starches and fats. Wonderful breads are ubiquitous across world cultures, and I can't imagine why anyone who can tolerate gluten proteins would want to avoid them. The challenge is not to overeat. For this, avoiding ultraprocessed foods might help.

But why do low-carb advocates think science is biased against them? If we ignore alcohol, our diets contain only three sources of calories: protein, carbohydrates, and fat. In any diet, protein intake doesn't vary by much, which leaves us with the other two sources: if carbs are low, fat has to be high. In the 1950s, studies linked saturated fats to higher blood cholesterol levels and to heart disease. Foods from animals are higher in saturated fatty acids than foods from plants.

Politics again. Advice to eat less meat elicited furious objections from that industry, which is especially powerful in the United States. Cattle are raised in every state, every state has two senators, and every senator is the target of meat-industry lobbyists. Today, the meat industry forges alliances with low-carb proponents to argue for higher meat intake. Politics does indeed make strange bedfellows.

Low-carb versus low-fat? I don't think it matters. What does matter are the calories, the foods they come from, and how processed those foods might be. Ultraprocessed foods tend to be high in sugars, refined carbs, and fats and, therefore, calories. We easily overeat them. The more we overeat, the more calories we take in, and the greater our risk for obesity and its health consequences.

Avoiding high-carb junk foods and sugary drinks is good advice for everyone, as is not gorging on red meats and fried foods. But if saying no to bread and pasta keeps you from overloading on calories, go for it. Omnivore that I am, I prefer diets with as few restrictions as possible, not least because cutting out either carbs or fats greatly detracts from the pleasures of eating. I'm for eating anything and everything—in moderation, of course.

4 CAN FOOD BE ADDICTIVE?

Kerry: Why do we overeat? Often, it's because we're stressed or depressed. Then there are the social gatherings; with so much temptation, who can resist sampling everything?

We're hardwired to crave sugars (and maybe fats) because they were the best sources of energy for our hunter-gatherer ancestors, who had to contend with far more unreliable food sources than we do. So, our metabolisms are a few centuries behind. The other taste we crave, salt, is an acquired taste. And oh, how we've acquired it!

But one aspect of this problem seems beyond our control: food companies that intentionally formulate their foods to reward the pleasure receptors in our brains. Of course food should be a pleasure to eat. But designing highly processed food products to trigger the release of dopamine, which is the same neurotransmitter that makes drugs like cocaine and methamphetamine so addictive? That goes beyond simply making foods taste good. Isn't it downright predatory?

Marion: It shouldn't surprise you or anyone else that food companies design products to make us want to eat them. That's their job. Their first priority is to return profits to shareholders. The more products we buy, the higher their profits. If we can't eat just one, they do better. And when the health consequences of obesity become collateral damage, that's our problem, not theirs. Food companies get to externalize those costs; we the people cover them. I view "addiction" to food products as just one more externalized cost of our current economic and food systems, right up there with greenhouse gas emissions and toxic algal blooms in the Gulf of Mexico. Business imperatives drive these systems. Is externalizing such costs fair or ethical? The answer depends entirely on your point of view.

I put addiction in quotation marks because I'm not convinced it correctly describes our relationship to foods we love to eat. It is one thing to enjoy a food but quite another to feel that survival and mental health depend on it. I hear all the time from people who feel this kind of dependence; some are under treatment for it. They tell me they crave specific foods—chocolate leaps to mind—or food in general. They obsess about the foods they crave, can't stop eating them, and fear that this obsession is ruining their lives.

Neuroscientists tell us that food triggers the same pleasure centers that respond to opioids, cigarettes, and alcohol, although not nearly to the same degree. While they and behavioral scientists are trying to sort out whether food cravings meet precise definitions of addiction, some food "addicts" tell me they are helped by twelve-step programs.

The quotation marks express my discomfort about using "addiction" to describe loving relationships to food. We can't live without eating. Food is delicious; eating it is a pleasure. Food companies cannot entice us to buy products that fail to trigger our brain's pleasure centers. Hence, as Michael Moss so compellingly explains in his book *Salt, Sugar, Fat,* food companies exploit our delight in those particular components to make products we want to buy.

It's too bad for us that the principal sources of salt, sugar, and fat in American diets are salty snack foods, sugary soft drinks, and fatty fried foods, respectively, all of them ultraprocessed junk foods deliberately formulated to make it hard for us to stop eating them.

You don't believe this? We now have the evidence for just how hard this is. People eating ultraprocessed foods are likely to eat more calories and—no surprise—gain weight. We know this from a clinical trial run by Kevin Hall and his colleagues at the National Institutes of Health. They managed to convince twenty adults to live in a controlled metabolic ward for a month. They gave the volunteers one of two diets—unprocessed or ultraprocessed—that were matched for calories, fat, carbohydrates, protein, and fiber. For two weeks, the volunteers could eat as much as they wanted of the assigned diet; they then could eat as much as they wanted of the other diet for two weeks. The results were stunningly clear, something that rarely happens in this kind of research. On the ultraprocessed diet, the volunteers consumed many more calories—500 more a day—than when eating the unprocessed diet. They also gained a pound a week.

How could something like this be possible? The volunteers did not realize they were eating more calories, and the scientists can only speculate. Pleasure centers in the brain are one possibility, and eating more quickly is another. But this experiment tells us that there is something about sweet, salty, and fatty foods that makes us want to eat more of them—and to be unaware of how much more we are eating. Salads and fruits do not trigger this kind of response. When we eat them and other relatively unprocessed foods, enough is enough. But hamburgers, fries, and a Coke? Not a chance.

We can argue forever about who holds responsibility for food choices, and whether these are matters of personal responsibility or are a result of the food environment. I think both, but I am endlessly surprised by the invisibility of the food industry as an influence on food choice. When I search Web images for "influences on obesity," I find plenty of diagrams mentioning family and peers or concerns about health, religion, or cost. Food-industry marketing? Not there. When marketing is done well, it is invisible. We are not supposed to notice the sales pitch when Beyoncé drinks Pepsi, and we don't.

Food companies spend billions of dollars in the United States and everywhere else to convince customers to buy their products, but as a marketing executive once explained to me, advertising is supposed to slip below the radar of critical thinking. In any case, advertising is just the tip of the iceberg. Food companies also promote their products through grocery store slotting fees, online games, music and sports entertainment, contributions to community groups, and, of course, research to find out what stimulates your pleasure centers so you will buy their products and come back for more.

Is this unethical? Not in our current economic system. Food companies are *supposed* to be doing all they can to maximize sales. They and their executives and stockholders are rewarded accordingly. To expect food companies to care about public health is to misunderstand their purpose. Eating more is good for business; eating less is not.

So where does that leave us? If you feel addicted to junk foods, you need all the help you can get. I sometimes eat junk food myself (no comments on that, please). Knowing how easy it is to eat too much of it, I buy it in small packages. If I know I will have trouble stopping once I start eating it, I try to keep it out of the house. It takes firm discipline to maintain this level of personal responsibility, and doing so is not fun. Eating healthfully would be easier if we didn't have junk food pushed at us constantly. It would help to have a more supportive food environment.

For this, we need an investment system that accepts lower profits in exchange for making health a priority. Until our culture adopts such values, we are on our own to navigate today's "eat more" food environment. Here's an alternative: let's advocate for a food environment that makes the healthy choice the easy choice, thereby helping us to have a healthier relationship with the foods we eat.

5 IS FAKE MEAT BETTER FOR US—AND THE PLANET—THAN THE REAL THING?

Kerry: I enjoy a nice, juicy steak as much as the next deeply conflicted carnivore. After all, eating too much meat is bad for us, bad for the environment, and definitely bad for the animals we slaughter to satisfy our carnivorous cravings.

Now we have Silicon Valley start-ups making veggie burgers that are so "impossibly" meat-like that they even "bleed." Millions of Americans who'd never dream of actually going vegetarian are suddenly showing a willingness to try soy and pea protein-based alternatives to a real burger.

In theory, this sounds like a win-win: less meat consumption! More ways to incorporate plants into your daily diet! But the more I learn about the way these imposter patties are produced, and some of the players who are involved in their production, the more perplexed I get. Are they really any better for us or the environment?

Marion: Investors have poured so much cash into plant-based meat alternatives—the brilliantly named Beyond Burger and Impossible Burger, for example—that I consider them the poster children for twenty-first-century food capitalism in action. Their admirers say these meat alternatives solve many of the problems caused by industrial animal production: they do not harm animals, induce antibiotic resistance, promote chronic disease, or produce as much greenhouse gas. Never mind reforming the system to raise food animals more humanely and sustainably. Food technologists can make more or less nutritionally equivalent analogs that don't involve animals, make people feel good about eating them, and sell at great profit.

No question, those of us in industrialized societies with the means to do so are eating too much meat for our own good or that of the planet. Dietary recommendations to promote planetary health list "eat less meat" as a major goal. Although some impoverished populations might be better off eating *more* meat—animal foods are good sources of nutrients that are missing or less readily available from other foods—most of us would do just fine eating less.

We Americans can and should be critical of how meat production methods affect animal health, our health, and the health of our environment, and be more aware of the ethical issues they raise. Those of us with adequate resources have the luxury of choosing whether to eat less meat, consume a largely plant-based diet, or go vegan and never eat animal foods at all. I eat meat, but not much, enjoy eating vegetables, and don't miss meat when I'm not eating it. Because I think it makes physiological sense to consume foods we evolved to eat, and I happen to prefer the taste of real foods, one of my personal food rules is never to eat anything artificial. I have a hard time understanding why anyone would want to eat fake anything, let alone concoctions that pretend to be meat.

But people who choose to be vegan for ethical reasons—they don't want animals killed or the environment destroyed—tell me they miss eating hamburgers, cheese, and ice cream and wish they had more food options. They insist that I be more open-minded about plant-based alternatives. I hear them, and am trying.

My first question: How do these products taste? As

soon as I could, I went to a high-end Manhattan restaurant to try its impossibly expensive Impossible Burger. The patty looked like beef but was so doused in ketchup that I couldn't really tell what I was eating. In the summer of 2019, I went to a specialty food show in New York for the express purpose of tasting every plant-based meat or dairy substitute I could find. To my palate, the fake meats came pretty close to the real thing in appearance, flavor, and texture, but were a lot saltier than I like. The plant-based cheeses were another matter; to me, they tasted gritty and need more work.

Meat and dairy alternatives do not fully duplicate the nutritional value of the animal-based originals, but I don't see that as a concern. Americans are hardly nutrient deprived; we are drowning in vitamins from fortified foods and get plenty more from everything else we eat. But I am concerned about how these things are made. Plant-based meats are decidedly ultraprocessed. They are industrially produced and full of ingredients never found in home kitchens, as witnessed by the ingredient list of a Beyond Burger:

Pea-protein isolate, expeller-pressed canola oil, refined coconut oil, contains 2% or less of the following: cellulose from bamboo, methylcellulose, potato starch, natural flavor, maltodextrin, yeast extract, salt, sunflower oil, vegetable glycerin, dried yeast, gum arabic, citrus extract (to protect quality), ascorbic acid (to maintain color), beet juice extract (for color), acetic acid, succinic acid, modified food starch, annatto (for color).

No, I did not make this up. Beyond Burgers taste salty because each patty contains nearly a gram, and even more salt comes with the toppings and bun.

Grant you, plant-based burgers have two things going for them: they do not require animals to be killed, and they have less saturated fat than beef. But pea protein? Protein of any kind is a non-issue in American diets; it is widely distributed in foods and most of us eat twice as much as we need. Even vegans should have no trouble meeting protein needs if they get enough calories and eat legumes—beans and peas. Extraction of the protein, however, leaves other legume nutrients behind.

Artificially constructed as they are, plant-based burgers are off my dietary radar. Vegetarian and vegan parents tell me they are relieved and thrilled to be able to take their kids to fast-food restaurants that serve these burgers, but to me they look like any other ultra-processed food. They raise the question of whether a better-for-you option is necessarily a *good* choice. Are these products really better for health than an occasional burger from pasture-raised beef? I have heard that studies to answer this question are under way and I look forward to seeing their results.

The jury is also still out on the benefits for climate change. I've seen comparisons and can pretty much guess who did them by what they report. People who favor these products find benefits; the industrial meat industry disagrees. So do people involved in small-scale animal agriculture, who point out that because ruminants can digest grasses that humans cannot, it is ecologically beneficial to graze them on land unusable for farming. Sustainable—what we are now calling "regenerative"—agriculture means replenishing nutrients and other valuable components in soil; for that, we need animal manure. It is surely better to use less land to grow feed for animals, and to avoid using all the fertilizers, pesticides, and herbicides feed crops require, but I'd like to see better data on the extent to which plant-based meats save water and land and reduce greenhouse gases. I am all for eating less meat, but less does not have to mean none.

If I am going to eat meat, I want it to come from animals raised as humanely and ecologically as possible. I like eating plant foods and I don't mind—and can afford—to pay a higher price for grass-fed beef or genuinely free-range chicken. I also know people who are more than willing to pay a higher price for plant-based dairy and meat alternatives; they view these products as making it possible for them to eat the same foods as everyone else and keep their ethical standards intact. Their point: anything is better than killing animals. My point: as long as the price of these products remains high, the choice of whether to consume them is an issue of class.

At the moment, I see these plant-based alternatives as wonders of food technology, techno-fixes for dealing with the much more complicated health, environmental, socioeconomic, and moral issues raised by industrial farm animal production. Nevertheless, I will be tracking the marketing of these products with great interest. I am also interested to see the public reaction to the next iteration of these products: laboratory-based meats created from cultured muscle cells.

These are not yet on the market, but investors are betting that they will be, and soon.

Are meat alternatives a fad? I think not. Vegetarians appreciate them. Eating less meat is good for health, the environment, and animal welfare. Big Meat companies such as Tyson, Perdue, and even Cargill have jumped into this market, as have fast-food chains. Sales are booming. I'm guessing that despite their socioeconomic and ultraprocessed contradictions, these products are here to stay—at least for those of us who can afford them.

6 IS IT A GOOD IDEA TO SELF-MEDICATE WITH SUPPLEMENTS OR SUPERFOODS?

Kerry: Sometimes I think pill-popping might be our true national pastime. Along with the dizzying array of over-the-counter and prescription drugs we down daily to treat our aches and pains, insomnia, constipation, depression, allergies, and a million other maladies, we're gobbling up gazillions of vitamins, supplements, fortified foods and so-called superfoods in our eternal quest for optimal wellness.

Should we take all these hyperbolic claims with a grain of salt? Maybe Himalayan pink salt, for which some people are willing to pay a premium because it gets its rosy hue from beneficial trace minerals such as potassium, magnesium, and calcium?

I find myself choosing certain foods because they're high in omega-3s, or antioxidants, or other reportedly beneficial phytochemicals. And I'm only too happy to bestow superpowers on my morning cup of coffee. Enhances memory! Improves physical performance! Lowers risk of stroke! But what if fish oil is just the new snake oil?

Marion: Magical thinking! As far as I can tell, humans must be hardwired to believe in nutritional magic. How else to explain why anyone would seriously believe that a pill is better than food, that vitamin-fortified ultra-processed foods are better than foods we evolved to eat, and that "superfoods" are better for health than any other food in the same group? These claims call for faith and wishful thinking. We believe in them despite an almost complete lack of evidence that they do much to improve the health of otherwise reasonably healthy people.

Supplements are a case in point. They come in two broad categories: nutrients and herbals (for want of a better term). Nutrients are easier to understand. They mainly include vitamins and minerals, but also other essential food components such as omega-3s and certain amino acids. The magic comes from thinking that if some are essential for health, more must be better. Alas, that's not how nutrition works. We need only minuscule amounts of vitamins. Eating a wide variety of relatively unprocessed foods usually takes care of nutrient needs and keeps the nutrients in balance.

The real magic is in the herbals: echinacea for colds, chondroitin for sore knee joints, kombucha for anything that ails you. Do people really believe that these work? Apparently so.

Magical thinking is the only reason I can think of to explain why more than half of American adults take dietary supplements despite overwhelming evidence that benefits, if any, are small, few do better than placebos, and some are harmful. Mind you, the absence of scientific support for supplements is not for lack of trying. The supplement industry is infamous for funding studies that show benefits for its products, but studies funded by independent sources rarely do. As I see it, the more rigorously studies of supplements are designed, the less benefit they show. But lack of scientific proof stops nobody from taking these products. As one devoted supplement taker assured me, "I don't care what the science says."

Granted, people who take supplements feel better taking them. In today's "eat more" food environment, dietary angst is a given. Every one of us has minor health complaints, and if a supplement might make us feel better, why not give it a try? We do. We feel better. Problem solved. This, however, is not science.

So what? Even if supplements only act as placebos, isn't that a benefit? And most dietary supplements are harmless, or less harmful than many pharmaceutical drugs. But exceptions exist, and the problem is knowing what those are. I cannot decide whether supplement makers genuinely believe in the benefits of their products or are just cynical about human nature. Whatever their motivation, they have used every trick in the book to win the right to market any supplement they want, in any way they want, with virtually no government oversight.

For this, we must thank Senator Orrin Hatch from Utah, where supplements are a big industry. He convinced Congress to essentially deregulate these products by passing the industry-written Dietary Supplement Health and Education Act (DSHEA) of 1994. This act assumes, not always correctly, that supplements are harmless. If the FDA disagrees, it has to take the supplement maker to court. DSHEA hampers FDA oversight so effectively that you cannot be sure that supplements are safe or labeled correctly. Studies have found supplement products with unlabeled drug ingredients, none of the labeled active ingredient, or other such inconsistencies.

Even worse, DSHEA undermines the FDA's ability to regulate health claims on foods, with unintended consequences for, of all things, interpretation of the First Amendment of the U.S. Constitution. DSHEA permits supplements to be marketed with "structure/function" claims—that a supplement promotes a healthy heart or bones, or improves cognitive function, for example—without requiring much in the way of scientific substantiation. This puts the FDA in an absurd position, forcing it to permit dubious "qualified" health claims to which it then adds a mind-boggling disclaimer: "FDA has determined that the evidence for this claim is limited and not conclusive."

Once the supplement industry was allowed to make such claims, food companies thought they should be allowed to use them too. They argued that health claims, backed by science or not, were allowed under First Amendment rights to free speech. I cannot believe that the founding fathers intended this amendment to protect the rights of food marketers to make misleading health claims, but the courts have repeatedly ruled in their favor, and the FDA eventually gave up fighting such cases. Today, the FDA avoids dealing with supplements except when claims or contents are flagrantly egregious. Supplements are the Wild West of the supermarket. Caveat emptor.

This leaves us with magical thinking to explain why we so easily fall for health claims on food products. Eating a fortified breakfast cereal will reduce our risk for heart disease? Pomegranate juice will prevent Alzheimer's? Microscopic amounts of minerals will make salt healthier? Even a moment's reflection ought to induce profound skepticism, but permission to say such things is a marketer's dream, and marketers pay for much of the research aimed at promoting such claims. When I see the title of a study claiming that mangos or cashews—as opposed to any other fruit or nut—do fabulous things for health, I can guess which trade association paid for it.

"Vitamins added" and "100% Daily Value" are highly effective selling points and are good examples of what the Australian sociologist Gyorgy Scrinis calls "nutritionism"—reducing the overall value of a food to its content of one or another nutrient. When General Mills advertises Chocolate Chex breakfast cereal as having more iron than black beans, it is using nutritionism to sell its product. The soda industry has long pressed the

FDA to allow it to add vitamins to products like Coke and Pepsi so it could market sugary drinks as healthy. To date, the FDA has resisted—its fortification policy prevents companies from adding vitamins to carbonated beverages. Companies get away with adding vitamins to sugar-sweetened waters and sports drinks because these drinks are not carbonated. Do Americans need more vitamins? Mostly no.

When I say anything about "superfoods" I use quotation marks, because this term has no nutritional meaning. It is a marketing term used to promote sales of specific fruits, vegetables, or nuts, most often for their antioxidant content. All plant foods contain antioxidants; by this definition, *all* are superfoods. Science, alas, shows little benefit (and, perhaps, harm) from antioxidant supplements. Plant foods are healthy and I'm all for promoting them, but is anyone really better off eating walnuts than any other nut, or grapes rather than any other fruit? I don't think so.

Supplements, fortified foods, and "superfoods" are about marketing, not science. Are fruits, vegetables, nuts, and whole grains good for you? Of course they are. But variety is a major nutrition principle—for reasons of pleasure as well as health.

II

THE COMMUNITY POLITICS OF FOOD CHOICE

7 WHY SHOULD ANYONE GO HUNGRY, EVER?

Kerry: Intractable social problems are like zombies; we whack away at them, but they just keep coming at us. How can such an affluent nation, blessed with abundant natural and human resources, have such high levels of homelessness and hunger?

The underlying causes of homelessness seem pretty obvious: a lack of affordable housing; ill-conceived housing policies; insufficient treatment options for substance abuse and mental illness; gentrification; racism; NIMBYism. The factors are easily named, if not easily solved.

But hunger, in the U.S.A., in the twenty-first century? That's got me totally stumped. You usually can't blame it on food shortages when our industrialized system of agriculture produces enough to feed everyone twice the number of calories they need on a daily basis.

Why should any child, woman, or man in this country ever go hungry? A distribution problem? Social inequality on steroids? Why can't we fix this?

Marion: Fix social inequality? Ask people at the top to pay higher taxes for a safety net that benefits everyone? Use taxpayer funds for affordable housing, public transportation, child care, universal school meals, health care, and public education (including college)? This sounds positively un-American in today's political climate. Our society expects us to take care of all that on our own. Too bad for you if you are born into a family with limited resources and limited opportunities.

Europeans pay somewhat, but not outrageously, higher taxes than we do, but look at what they get in return—all that and more. They are beyond shocked at what we have to pay for health care and higher education, and they pity us for it. Convincing Americans to be willing to pay higher taxes for social purposes would require strong leadership from everyone from the president and Congress on down. Some members of Congress, particularly the newer ones, get this. Let's make sure they grow in number. We won't solve the hunger problem without them.

I was born into a poor family during the Great Depression, but we must have scraped by because I don't remember going hungry except between meals. I observed hunger and homelessness first hand when I was in public health school in the mid-1980s and did my year-long fieldwork with San Francisco's Coalition of Homeless Shelter Providers. Reagan-era cuts to social programs had left many people destitute and food insecure—lacking reliable food on a daily basis. City and state surveys at the time made two things clear: food stamp benefits ran out before the end of the month (as they still do), and private sector efforts to fill the gap could not come close to meeting the need (as they still do not).

I volunteered in soup kitchens run by St. Anthony's and the Episcopal Sanctuary. We did the best we could with donations, but these seemed haphazard and less than ideal for improving the lives of the people we served, many of them newly released from mental institutions, addicted to alcohol or drugs, or shell-shocked veterans. Soup kitchens do much better now, and the demographic has shifted. Today's hungry and homeless increasingly include victims of rising rents, unaffordable health care, and plain bad luck, many of them women and children. We could solve this problem with better education, jobs, affordable housing, and supportive mental health and social services. Countries that do these things have reduced needs for such services. The United States is rich enough to do this too. But the private sector alone can never—and will not—fill the need. Dealing with hunger and homelessness is what government is supposed to do.

What's lacking, obviously, is political will. We have become inured to the hungry and homeless. When we resent panhandlers on the street or in the subway and blame them for their own plight, we join a long tradition dating back to the English Poor Laws of the 1600s. Instead of viewing the destitute as victims of rapidly changing economic systems or other circumstances beyond their control, the Poor Laws viewed those without means as inherently unworthy and poverty as a matter of personal choice. The laws assumed that poor people could educate themselves and get well-paying jobs if they really wanted to. Then as now, politicians feared that any assistance would induce dependency on tax-supported handouts. The laws provided just enough aid to keep people from dying on the streets (inconvenient, unsightly) or engaging in outright rebellion (politically problematic), but never enough to live decently. Although ostensibly aimed at relieving hunger, the Poor Laws also had political purposes: keep the destitute off the streets and willing to work for low wages.

Today's politicians still use welfare and food assistance for these purposes but add one more: they gain power by exploiting the poor. We see this play out in congressional debates about SNAP (the Supplemental Nutrition Assistance Program), formerly known as food stamps. The debates focus entirely on how to reduce SNAP enrollments and costs, never on how best to bring people out of poverty. Many SNAP participants hold jobs but are paid so little that they qualify for federal food assistance. When employees of Walmart and Amazon must rely on SNAP to get by, as many do, we taxpayers enable corporations to perpetuate poverty.

SNAP is the largest of the federal food assistance programs. It is an entitlement, like Medicare and Social Security, and one of the last vestiges of what used to be a much stronger safety net. Its benefits are convincingly documented, but the program could do even better. In 2018, SNAP cost taxpayers $65 billion in benefits and administrative costs, but with more than 40 million participants, the average monthly benefit was just $125. This amount goes further in rural areas, where plenty of poverty exists, and it helps even in urban areas, but it is nowhere near enough to get people on their feet.

I wish SNAP benefits were greater—much greater—but I also wish SNAP did more to promote healthy food choices. As it is, SNAP benefits are spent mostly at grocery stores, where recipients can choose pretty much whatever foods they like. Choice is good, but grocery stores are deliberately designed to push sales of the most highly profitable ultraprocessed foods, making SNAP a program that promotes the financial health of retailers more than the health of its recipients. Low-income and segregated neighborhoods often don't have grocery stores, limiting choices to whatever bodegas or convenience stores can offer.

I wish our society paid more attention to how best to address the food needs of people who don't have much money, not least because the cost of fruits and vegetables has risen so much more than the cost of ultraprocessed foods. We should be deep in discussion about how best to raise living standards. We should seriously consider methods used in other countries: cash transfers, universal basic incomes, and subsidized child care, housing, education, and health care. Or we could address two problems at once: subsidize small farmers for growing food sold to poor people at low cost. But even a conversation about such possibilities requires political will.

For reasons of history—and lack of political will—advocates have no choice but to focus on protecting SNAP from further cuts. If we had a chance to start over on policies to address hunger, we might be able to consider better options. In the meantime, we have hungry mouths to feed, and half of SNAP recipients are children. Don't we have some responsibility to help them? I think we do. And yes, I see this as a government responsibility. As Janet Poppendieck eloquently described in her 1998 book *Sweet Charity*, we currently run a parallel food system for feeding the poor that includes thousands of volunteer food banks, food pantries, and soup kitchens. No matter how good they are—and many are remarkably effective—they are too dependent on private donations to provide a secure safety net for the hungry people they serve.

If my time on the front lines of anti-hunger advocacy taught me anything, it is that private-sector programs are not a long-term solution. For that we need public policy, meaning laws and regulations authorizing tax-payer funds to bring people out of poverty. I worry that private-sector approaches keep the people who are running these programs so hard at work to meet their clients' immediate needs for food that neither they nor the people they serve have the bandwidth to get involved in what is really needed—massive civil society demand for policies to reduce hunger, food insecurity, homelessness, as well as to address the economic and societal inequalities responsible for these conditions.

8 IS OBESITY REALLY ONLY A MATTER OF PERSONAL RESPONSIBILITY?

Kerry: No one intentionally overfills the gas tank in their car, presumably because there's a shut-off mechanism that prevents us from over-pumping. Sadly, no such mechanism exists to stop us from routinely overfilling our bellies. And if we habitually take in more fuel than we burn, it's bound to add fat to our frames. But, like many other Americans who are now overweight or obese, I ignore this simple equation.

I know I need to develop greater impulse control, but our culture actively promotes, and even celebrates, overeating. Portions are absurdly large. We snack all day. Candy and sodas have been around for more than a century but used to be considered a special treat. Now, they're at virtually every checkout counter. We're only human! Now that corporations have been legally declared to be people too, shouldn't they take pity on us and stop encouraging us to overfuel?

Marion: Think of what we are up against. We have to eat, and food is available everywhere at prices most of us can afford. I'm sure some people can resist, but I too have a hard time refusing food I like when it is right in front of me. When I was a kid, the food environment was a lot different. In poor families like mine, there wasn't much extra food around. We ate at mealtimes. Too bad for us if we were hungry between meals. My friends and I were expected to play outside until dinner was served. If we were thirsty, we turned on the tap or found a public water fountain. I went to public schools in largely white, lower-middle-class neighborhoods where an occasional kid might be overweight—and teased mercilessly for it—but for most of us, weight was not an issue.

Then came the 1980s. Suddenly, everyone seemed to develop a weight problem. The average weight of Americans increased by fifteen to twenty pounds between 1980 and 2000. Clothing sizes grew bigger to accommodate bigger people; waistbands became elastic. How did this happen? Americans were eating more food—300 to 500 more calories every day, on average.

It takes three to five miles of walking or running to compensate for that many calories. At the same time, work and play were becoming less physically demanding. No wonder so many people gained weight.

As the co-author of a book called *Why Calories Count,* I obviously think calorie balance matters. If you eat more calories than you use, you will gain weight. Some overeaters gain more weight more quickly than others, perhaps because of genetics, the foods the calories come from, or even the microbiome. But everyone who overeats calories gains weight.

Why were people eating more calories? Genetics did not change, and neither did food preferences, our sense of personal responsibility, or our microbiomes. What did change was the food environment—the physical and social context in which we make food choices. Suddenly, food was available everywhere, any time, and in much larger amounts.

Consider how this happened. As I see it, the food environment changed in the early 1980s as the result of policy shifts in three areas: agriculture, Wall Street, and food regulation. The agricultural changes started in the 1970s. Before then, the government paid farmers to leave part of their land unplanted as a way to prevent overproduction, thereby keeping prices high enough for them to make a living. But then came Earl Butz, who as USDA secretary advised and subsidized farmers to grow as much food as they possibly could. More acres planted meant more food produced; more production meant more calories. Between 1980 and 2000, the number of calories available in the U.S. food supply per capita—amounts produced, plus imports, less exports—went from about 3,200 per day to 4,000, about twice the number of calories most people need. Even if, as the USDA maintains, one-third of those calories is wasted, they are still in surplus. Now food companies had to compete harder to sell products in a hugely overabundant marketplace.

Why Wall Street? The shareholder value movement came into its own in the early 1980s. This movement rejected blue-chip stocks that produced low but reliable returns on investment (IBM is the classic example). Instead, its followers demanded higher and more immediate returns on their investments. Making a profit was no longer enough. Companies now had to continuously increase their profits to keep stock prices high. Continuous growth is challenging for all corporations, but especially so for food companies; they were already trying to sell products in a marketplace teeming with excess calories.

Food companies responded by developing new products (enticing consumption), making more food available outside the home (where people tend to eat more calories), increasing the number of fast-food restaurants (where food is highly caloric and cheap), and promoting snacking (more calories). They put food where it had never been sold before: in drugstores, clothing stores, office supply stores, bookstores, libraries. The deregulatory policies of the Reagan administration allowed companies to market more aggressively to children, and they increasingly targeted their marketing to marginalized groups, racial and ethnic minorities, and populations in low-income countries.

These changes also explain the influx of larger serving sizes. Because overabundant food is cheap (an issue of supply versus demand), companies could introduce big portions at little additional cost. I remember when giant 600-calorie muffins first appeared in the late 1980s, replacing what are now considered mini muffins (200 calories). If I could communicate just one nutritional concept, it would be this: larger portions have more calories!

As my NYU colleague Lisa Young has shown in her research, the rise in obesity tracks closely with the introduction of larger portion sizes. The giant sizes have especially affected sugary drinks, snack foods, and fast foods—the ultraprocessed foods we can't stop eating—as well as restaurant portions.

All of this makes it evident why overweight and obesity are so much more prevalent among people with scarce resources. Ultraprocessed foods are cheap in large amounts. Food companies market directly to low-income groups, making sure that their products are readily available in any corner store, taste good, are convenient, and sell at prices anyone can afford. For such marketing campaigns, health consequences are irrelevant.

Resisting today's food environment is not for the faint-hearted. I think it helps to pay attention to marketing techniques. Critical thinking also helps, and examining weight-loss "miracles" is a good place to begin. For a diet to work, it has to help you eat less. Most diets do this by restricting whole categories of foods—the current favorite is carbohydrates. If you avoid eating sugars, sugary drinks, donuts, bread, rice, pasta, pizza, and the like, you will not be consuming the calories they provide. If you don't compensate by eating huge portions of hamburgers and fries, the pounds ought to fall off without your even noticing. I did not intend *Soda Politics* to be a diet book, but after its publication I received any number of letters from people telling me that when they stopped drinking sodas, their weights dropped—by ten, twenty, forty, and in one case, eighty pounds. Cutting out sodas cuts calories.

Wouldn't it be terrific if we could fix the food environment so that it makes the healthy choice the easier, and the less expensive, choice? For that, we need politics. How about advocating for rules that make it easier to eat smaller amounts—for example, setting standards for the size of food portions, giving a price break for smaller portions, or putting calorie limits on restaurant portions. How about restricting food-industry marketing, especially of ultraprocessed foods, and especially marketing targeted at kids? Without that kind of help, you had best gear up your personal responsibility skills. You will need them every minute to navigate today's food marketing environment.

9 WHY ISN'T HEALTHY SCHOOL FOOD A NO-BRAINER?

Kerry: Our politicians often cite their fervent desire to "create a better future" for the next generation. If only that noble vision truly motivated them to use their legislative powers to benefit all our children, regardless of race, class, region, religion, or any other category that might foster marginalization.

The way that politicians allocate resources and establish guidelines for the National School Lunch Program suggests that universal healthy school lunches are a much lower priority than funneling government aid to industrialized agriculture. How else to explain the eternal reluctance to rethink agricultural and nutritional policies that actually encourage childhood obesity and diabetes?

Surely it would be less expensive in the long run to provide adequate funding to feed all our children well?

Why isn't it a no-brainer to pass policies that nourish school kids with wholesome, nutritious lunches?

Marion: The short answer: money and politics. You and I might view school food as an issue that unites everyone across the entire political spectrum. Doesn't everyone want schools to give kids the nutritional power they need to become strong, smart, and effective adults? Apparently not.

Recall what happened to Michelle Obama's Let's Move campaign. In 2010, the then–first lady took on childhood obesity as her personal cause. I was thrilled that someone in the White House actually cared about the same food issues I did. I thought her focus on school food was terrific but wondered if the first lady knew what she was taking on. Did she think school food would be a nonpartisan issue that schools, parents, and Congress could all rally behind? Or did she know right from the start that in advocating for healthier school food, she would have to confront the food industry about what it was selling to schools and marketing to kids?

To the extent she could, Michelle Obama did confront this industry, starting with encouraging Congress to pass the Healthy Hunger-Free Kids Act of 2010.

Because this act set nutrition standards for *all* foods served in schools, I wondered whether legislators had read its fine print. "All" included not only federally subsidized breakfasts and lunches, but also snacks and sodas sold outside of those meals. Once the USDA published its proposals for nutrition standards mandated by the act, I was not surprised that all hell broke loose.

Lobbyists swarmed Congress. Food companies spent millions to convince legislators to weaken the standards so their products could continue to be sold in schools. Potato trade associations and pizza suppliers spent even more millions to lobby against proposed limits on the number of times fried potatoes could be served in a week, and on the volume of tomato paste that qualified as a vegetable. This worked. You might think that Congress ought to have better things to do, but it directed the USDA to let schools serve French fries every day and count even a spoonful of tomato sauce on pizza as a serving of vegetables (I'm not making this up).

Once the USDA issued the final rules, the opposition became even louder, much of it from an unexpected source—the School Nutrition Association (SNA), which represents school food service personnel. The SNA had four complaints: school meal programs are underfunded (this one has merit), the kids don't like the food, the new standards cause more waste, and schools need more time to change their menus (these last three are contradicted by research). Taking up where food companies left off, the SNA leadership—against the will of much of its membership—lobbied Congress and the USDA, organized opposition to the standards, and paid for its own self-serving research. Why? It can hardly be a coincidence that 40 percent of the SNA's funding comes from companies that sell food products to schools.

Despite all this, school meals seem greatly improved. I visit schools every chance I get to see for myself what the meals look like, how they taste, and whether the kids are eating them. Thanks to dedicated food service workers, some schools run exemplary meal programs. The food smells good, the kids eat it, and not much goes into the garbage. In others, the food is just fine, but the kids aren't eating it. In still others, nothing works. The critical difference? The adults who run the program. If they care about feeding kids—and many do—it's a good bet that the food is edible and the kids are eating it.

But funding is a genuine barrier. Unlike any other public school program, meals are expected to be self-supporting. USDA reimbursements for the meals have to cover the cost of labor and supplies and leave barely enough for the food. Schools without kitchens must rely on more expensive pre-prepared meals. USDA payments depend on participation levels, but only some children are eligible for free or reduced-price meals, leading to heartbreaking problems of denial of benefits and stigmatization. One way to solve these problems would be to make school meals universal—free breakfasts and lunches for all children. New York City is doing this, to excellent effect. No child should ever go hungry. Universal school meals should be national policy.

Wherever possible, so should school gardens. In some of New York City's poorest neighborhoods, I've seen public school kids harvest salad greens from pots and planters, wash and prepare them, eat them, and ask for seconds. By this time, plenty of research shows that school gardens encourage kids to like and eat vegetables, and it would be wonderful if every school had one, even if only in pots on windowsills.

But can we do anything to stop the food industry from relentlessly marketing ultraprocessed products to kids in schools and at home? Michelle Obama tried.

She told food industry executives that they needed to entirely rethink the products they were offering and how they marketed their products to children. Brave words. But I once attended a White House meeting where food company representatives flatly drew the line at having to stop marketing to kids: "We have a fiduciary duty to our stockholders," they told us. From their standpoint, corporate profits had to come first; considerations of children's health were decidedly secondary.

I cannot fathom how school food has become a flash point for pushback over nanny-state overreach. Food companies are brilliant at exploiting parental insecurity about feeding kids. Anything that feels like a criticism of parenting practices adds to anxiety. If schools do not sell sodas and snacks, discourage teachers from rewarding kids with candy, and restrict cupcakes for birthday celebrations, some parents feel personally criticized and complain. Schools need to take such complaints seriously, explain why they want kids to eat more healthfully, and ask to be given a chance to demonstrate the value of creating a healthier food environment.

I wish there were an easy way for everyone connected with schools to see the bigger picture of junk food in schools. In her 2019 book *Kid Food,* Bettina Siegel tracks the astonishing amount of sweets given to kids in classes as treats or rewards for correct answers. One of our NYU doctoral students who worked in an elementary school could hardly believe what parents brought in for birthday celebrations. She added up the calories from cake, ice cream, candy, punch, or snacks: 250 to 450 per kid per celebration, and this for kindergarten kids, no less.

Schools need more money for school meals, and free or affordable meals should be universal. But it would be good if the meals were based on food, not food products, and kept ultraprocessed items to a minimum. Birthdays and other celebrations could be managed—limited to once a week or month—to minimize calories, especially from sugar. Gold stars for performance worked for me when I was a kid. Could we try something like that again? And as long as we get to dream about what might be ideal, let's make sure schools have functioning kitchens and gardens whenever they can, and teach kids to grow and prepare food. I've been in schools where all this is happening, and it is a beautiful thing to see. Kids in schools in neighborhoods rich and poor deserve this and more.

10 WHY DON'T WE DEMAND A HIGHER STANDARD OF FOOD SAFETY?

Kerry: There's no getting around the scary fact that eating the wrong thing can sicken or even kill us. Our food production system appears to be filled with all kinds of hazards, too.

We have plenty of regulations intended to protect consumers and workers. And yet, out in the fields, toxic pesticides and herbicides jeopardize the health of the farm workers who apply them, and the residues from these toxins may contaminate the produce itself. Slaughterhouses—notoriously dangerous places to work—put workers at great risk of injury and illness, due to crowding and ever-faster processing procedures.

Antibiotic overuse in livestock has rendered those antibiotics increasingly ineffective in humans, creating potentially deadly "superbugs." *E. coli* and *Salmonella* outbreaks regularly make the news. It seems as if there's so much potential for harm, from farm to table. Just how corroded is our food chain?

Marion: Food safety is a major national headache. We do have laws and regulations, and they are vastly better than they used to be. What we do not have is a committed food safety culture. By this I mean that everyone involved in producing a food, from the executive suite to the front lines at the packing plants, feels personally responsible for producing safe food and adheres to safety procedures—in spirit as well as in letter.

Thanks to NASA, we know how to produce safe food. Its officials knew that they could not risk having astronauts get food poisoning, especially under conditions of zero gravity. They devised a highly effective series of prevention controls: identify the places in food production where contamination can occur, take steps to prevent that from happening, and monitor to make sure those steps were effective. This method worked brilliantly in outer space and ought to work on Earth. That it doesn't is a travesty that puts lives at risk.

Judging by the daily recalls of foods contaminated with dangerous bacteria or chemicals, too many food producers seem to give lip service to food safety without internalizing it as a personal or corporate value. Why should they? If they slow the production lines, they don't make as much money. If they find a safety lapse, they may have to stop the line or recall products. These disincentives are so powerful that companies would rather conduct business as usual and risk the costs of worker injuries or an occasional illness outbreak. Even when corporate negligence is shown to cause workers to be hurt or eaters to become sick, hospitalized, or die, the consequences to the company are limited.

Where is government oversight? Its problems are legendary. The U.S. government deals with food safety through thirty different laws administered by fifteen federal agencies, of which two matter most: the USDA for meat and poultry, and the FDA for pretty much everything else—as if pathogenic bacteria excreted by farm animals never get anywhere near fields of vegetables. The Government Accountability Office has been complaining—for more than forty years, if you can believe it—about the lack of coordination between USDA and FDA oversight, so much so that it considers food safety to be a high-risk enterprise. As well it should: according to CDC estimates, about one in six Americans (48 million) is sickened by a foodborne

pathogen each year; more than 125,000 are hospitalized and 3,000 die.

In 2019, nearly 200 people became ill from eating
pork contaminated with a particularly nasty *Salmonella*
strain resistant to four antibiotics, but pork producers
refused to allow CDC investigators on their farms. They
do not have to. The meat industry's lobbying and campaign contributions ensure that company participation
in safety investigations is largely voluntary.

Why do we tolerate this? Lobbying and donations
to election campaigns are legal, but I'm guessing that
common experience explains the lack of outrage. Most
of us have had episodes of food poisoning at one time
or another. We felt awful for a day or two but then
recovered. Such episodes seem normal. Outrage only
comes when someone we care about dies from toxic *E.
coli* in a hamburger, *Salmonella* in eggs or peanut butter, or *Listeria* in soft cheeses. Only then do we join Stop
Foodborne Illness, an advocacy organization formed
by parents of children who died from eating contaminated Jack in the Box hamburgers in 1993. That company cleaned up its food safety procedures and has not
caused further illnesses, but food safety advocates still
have plenty of work to do. Getting sick from food should

never be considered normal, and advocates need far more support. So does the FDA. Congress has limited the FDA's oversight ability by expanding its responsibilities without keeping up with its funding needs.

Advocates do get support from food safety lawyer Bill Marler, who began his career representing Jack in the Box victims. He continues to work on behalf of victims of unsafe food to obtain hefty payments from negligent producers. When lawyers can show that a contaminated food makes someone sick, they win their cases. This makes the courts responsible for enforcing food safety laws—after the damage is done.

Preventive food safety regulations could be better coordinated, but food companies need to take the ones we have more seriously, and so do federal agencies. The otherwise preoccupied USDA and the resource-poor FDA can't do much about producers, so they shift responsibility for food safety to us eaters. They advise us to *clean* (wash hands and surfaces), *separate* (don't cross-contaminate), *cook* (to the right temperature), and *chill* (refrigerate promptly). This is always good advice, but wouldn't it be better to ensure that foods are safe when they get to us? We should not have to run our kitchens like maximum-security biological laboratories.

One factor in our favor: cooking kills most food pathogens. That is why Bill Marler says he never drinks raw water, milk, or juice, and never eats raw sprouts or shellfish, raw or undercooked meat, eggs, or flour, or prewashed or cut fruits and vegetables. The risk of illness from eating these foods may be small, but it is higher than that from cooked foods or those handled by fewer people. Is the risk worth it? That's up to you to decide.

You do not, however, have a choice about chemical contaminants. Our water and food supplies too often contain lead, toxic chemicals, and agricultural fertilizers, pesticides, and herbicides, usually in trace amounts but sometimes at levels above what is considered safe. Except for lead, which has no safe level, it's hard to say how harmful the others are to our health, in part because their manufacturers are so good at manufacturing doubt about their harm and lobbying Congress to stop independent research and government regulation. Here's one place where inequities in our food system are flagrantly obvious: poor communities are most at risk from contaminated soil and water, as we learned from the scandal over lead-contaminated tap water in Flint, Michigan—a problem still not adequately addressed.

Even when levels of chemical contaminants are considered safe, their presence in our food and water is not necessarily acceptable. I am unaware of evidence that any of these chemicals improves our health, and plenty of studies suggest otherwise. More research might help, but mostly we need better oversight, laws, and enforcement.

Monsanto's glyphosate—Roundup—is a prime example. This herbicide is applied in massive quantities to control weeds around genetically modified corn and soybeans and is also widely used by homeowners unaware that it might be hazardous. An international cancer research agency says glyphosate is probably carcinogenic and may raise the risk of non-Hodgkin's lymphoma. This chemical's current owner, Bayer (which bought Monsanto), insists that glyphosate is safe, but juries in several court cases have disagreed. While the safety of glyphosate is debated by scientific committees and the courts, it seems sensible to avoid it.

But how? The only way I know is to buy organic foods or those with non-GMO labels. The USDA's organic rules explicitly forbid use of the most harmful agricultural chemicals—reason enough to choose organic foods—and of genetic modification. If these foods are too expensive or unavailable, it's worth trying to avoid at least the ones that are most heavily contaminated—the Environmental Working Group's "Dirty Dozen," for example. In 2019, strawberries headed the list, followed by spinach, kale, nectarines, and apples. This group also publishes a list of the "Clean 15," foods most likely to be pesticide-free, including avocados, sweet corn, pineapples, peas, and onions.

Food safety, alas, is governed by politics more than public health. When tap water in Flint, in Newark, New Jersey, and in other neglected low-income cities is found to contain lead, this is a sure sign that the populations are disenfranchised and political leaders are not doing their job. If we get sick from eating contaminated eggs, hamburgers, or cheese, it means their producers are not adhering to food safety laws, and the USDA and FDA are not enforcing those laws adequately. This needs to change. Change means political action.

We need to speak out and demand that food companies take the safety of food—and food workers—seriously, that oversight agencies do the same, and that Congress gives these agencies the rules and resources they need to do their job. I would like to see food safety kept high on the agenda for food-system advocacy.

11 WHY CAN'T WE STOP WASTING FOOD?

Kerry: We live in an era of such abundance that we now throw away roughly 40 percent of the food we produce. How appalling is that? Sure, some food waste is inevitable. But at a time when 40 million people are on the Supplemental Nutrition Assistance Program (SNAP), why does the food industry discard six billion pounds of perfectly edible food annually because of minor physical imperfections or ambiguous, perplexing "sell by" dates?

We're not just wasting the actual food, but all the fossil fuels and water it took to produce it too. Adding insult to injury, the food waste we send to landfills generates methane gas as it rots, making climate change worse. Folks who lived through food shortages in the Depression and World War II treated food as a precious resource, which it was. Is there anything short of economic collapse or war that could bring back that mindset?

Marion: Waste is high on the food advocacy agenda right now. Preventing food waste is one of those actions—like contributing to food banks—that everyone can do and feel good about. In public health terms, encouraging people to stop wasting food is a "downstream" approach. It puts the burden on us as individuals to address problems in food and agriculture policies that happen long before food gets to us. We all could do a better job of using the food we buy, but that doesn't get at the real problem: too much food to begin with.

The "we" in your question implies that it's our fault so much food is wasted. If you and I weren't so fussy about how foods look, and retailers didn't have to toss out packages past their sell-by dates, we could distribute that food to those in need, reduce our impact on the environment, and create a big win-win for all.

Yes, we could, but USDA data say that we eaters are responsible for only 20 percent of food waste, and retailers for even less—10 percent. What retailers toss into dumpsters may be highly visible, but most retail waste goes to the makers of pet food or animal feed. Processors also do not waste much; they use misshapen fruits and vegetables for canned foods or sauces.

That leaves 70 percent of losses—the vast majority—

at the levels of production or harvest. For Americans, the waste problem begins with an overabundant food system—4,000 daily calories per capita, roughly one third of them wasted. Some of the 70 percent is the inevitable result of bad weather, insects, molds, or incomplete harvesting, but waste is built into our food system from the get-go.

I want more attention focused on that 70 percent. I did once attend a meeting of Champions 12.3, an organization of high-level international business executives committed to eliminating half the waste in their food supply chains by 2030 (the 12.3 refers to one of the United Nations' Sustainable Development Goals discussed in chapter 17). Food companies love to cite waste reduction as one of their sustainability initiatives—it's something they can achieve without threatening their bottom lines.

Once we start looking at overproduction as the root cause of food waste, we have to consider how agricultural support policies have led to having twice the number of calories in the food supply than our population actually needs. These policies do practically nothing to encourage organic vegetable production or regenerative farming methods but generously reward farmers for producing as much corn and soy as they possibly can, thereby encouraging these crops to be grown even on land where soils are poor or water insufficient.

Overproduction makes commodity crops—and the food products made from them—so cheap that we don't think twice about throwing them away. Overproduction explains why we have 50,000 or so products in an average supermarket, all-you-can-eat buffets, supersize portions, and prepared foods everywhere, many of them vulnerable to spoilage if kept around too long.

Confronted with so much food, we have two choices: eat it or waste it. If we eat it, we gain weight. Obesity is an externalized cost of overproduction, and an expensive one. Waste is another. The best we can do with wasted food is to divert it—to pet food, animal feed, compost, or as you suggest, to food banks. Otherwise, it ends up in landfills, produces methane, and adds to environmental degradation and climate change.

I have no trouble with the idea of using food waste to feed pets, but I firmly believe that humans deserve better. Food banks have become a parallel food distribution system that often must operate on the principle that anything is better than nothing. Most do the best they can with whatever food and cash they receive, and some do splendid work, but what they can offer too often comes down to highly processed foods with long shelf life. Cash donations must be stretched to meet needs, which often means skimping on fresh perishables.

I often hear pleas for more effective diversion to food banks of discarded foods from farms, supermarkets, college cafeterias, restaurants, and caterers. Organizations in nearly every city in America are working hard to do this, despite formidable safety and logistical challenges. I once visited an upstate New York farmer whose just-harvested fields were littered with melons, squash, and corn missed or rejected during harvesting. He had invited every food bank within driving distance to come glean his fields but none could manage the complications and cost of trucking and labor. All of us can and should do our part to buy only what we need and try to find uses for the waste for which we are responsible, but surely there are better ways to ensure that no American goes hungry.

If we really want to deal with food waste—and with food insecurity—we need to confront both problems at their source. For food waste, let's insist on agricultural policies that reward farmers for quality, conservation, and use of sustainable methods, not for how much they produce. Years ago, we had conservation restrictions on the amounts of food farmers could grow. These are worth considering again. In the meantime, let's help address poverty by paying decent wages to farm workers and assuring farmers a fair price for what they produce.

I am well aware that such measures would increase food costs. High quality food is more expensive to produce. The price of organic foods is higher than that of conventionally grown foods because organic production methods take more work. If industrialized food producers had to pay the externalized costs of their practices by cleaning up environmental pollution, replenishing soil, and managing waste, the cost of all food, not just organics, would be higher for everyone.

Some of us can afford to pay more for better food, and may well consider it worth the price. But where does that leave the tens of millions of Americans who barely get by as it is and would be pushed even deeper into poverty by higher food prices? This dilemma makes distribution of food waste seem attractive. Diverting discarded food to poor people helps solve an immediate problem but keeps everyone too busy to do what is really needed: organizing political power to reduce poverty and its causes.

As I hope is obvious by now, I see food waste as a much larger issue. Everyone everywhere needs governments to deal with both sides of the waste issue—preventing overproduction and composting what isn't used—but also to be doing all they can to reduce the class and social inequities that cause hunger in the first place. If governments were working to meet these responsibilities, it would be easier for all of us to respect food as the treasure it is.

12 DO WE NEED A NATIONAL FOOD POLICY AGENCY?

Kerry: We demand a lot from our government agencies. We want them to be there for us when disaster strikes or disease breaks out. We want policies that protect us from danger and help us lead healthy lives.

But what happens when an agency has multiple agendas that conflict? Like, for example, the USDA, whose mission is to help farmers turn a profit, while also promoting healthy eating habits. We end up with an agency whose agricultural policies actively encourage diseases that cost millions of lives and billions of dollars annually, even as its nutrition policies try to tackle those same largely preventable illnesses.

Academics, "good food" advocates, and health care experts have proposed that we break this vicious cycle by creating a national food policy agency that would adopt a more enlightened approach. Can you imagine such an agency?

Marion: Easily. I'm often asked what I would do if I were the boss of America's food system. High on my action list would be reorganizing federal food and nutrition policies to get them all focused on preventing hunger, promoting health, and protecting the environment. In the United States, we have plenty of policies dealing with these goals, but responsibility for them is fragmented among multiple agencies, each with its own political leadership, constituency, and policy agenda. Each competes with the others for mandates and funding. And each attracts its own dedicated horde of stakeholder lobbyists.

A list is all you need to understand why current policies seem at cross purposes. I can think of eleven distinct categories of policies for agriculture, food, and nutrition. The USDA is in charge of most of them, but not all, and some of its functions overlap with those of other agencies. I realize that a table oversimplifies this situation, but I think it's the easiest way to get a quick overview. See if you agree.

The explanation for a system this complicated is history—and politics, of course. The policies developed piecemeal, mostly during the twentieth century, in response to specific problems as they arose.

U.S. policy areas dealing with agriculture, food, and nutrition

POLICY AREA	MANDATE	OVERSIGHT AGENCY (OR AGENCIES)
Agricultural support	Payments to producers based on congressional farm bill legislation	USDA
Alcoholic beverages	Regulation of production, imports, labels, advertising	TTB
Environmental impact of food production and consumption	Standards for protecting quality of soil, water, and air; farmland conservation	USDA, EPA
Food and nutrition monitoring	Food quantity and quality, dietary intake, and effects of diets on health	USDA, CDC
Food and nutrition research	Studies of agriculture, food, nutrition, and health	NIH, USDA, FDA, CDC
Food assistance	Nutritional support for low-income adults and children through programs such as SNAP, WIC, and school meals	USDA

(*continued*)

POLICY AREA	MANDATE	OVERSIGHT AGENCY (OR AGENCIES)
Food labor	Regulation of working conditions for farm, slaughterhouse, and restaurant employees	U.S. Department of Labor (wages, working conditions, child labor, migrant and seasonal workers); USDA (surveys, statistics); OSHA (worker safety and health)
Food product regulation	Package contents, labels, health claims, advertising	USDA (meat and poultry); FDA (all other foods, supplements); FTC (advertising)
Food safety	Procedures, inspections, enforcement	USDA (meat and poultry); FDA (all other foods)
Food trade	Quality and safety standards for agricultural crop, food product, ingredient, and supplement imports and exports	USDA, FDA, and 20 other federal agencies
Nutrition education	Dietary Guidelines for Americans; MyPlate food guide	USDA and HHS (guidelines); USDA (MyPlate)

Abbreviations: CDC, Centers for Disease Control and Prevention; EPA, Environmental Protection Agency; FDA, Food and Drug Administration; FTC, Federal Trade Commission; NIH, National Institutes of Health; HHS, Department of Health and Human Services; OSHA, Occupational Safety and Health Administration; SNAP, Supplemental Nutrition Assistance Program; TTB, Alcohol and Tobacco Tax and Trade Bureau; USDA, U.S. Department of Agriculture; WIC, Special Supplemental Nutrition Program for Women, Infants, and Children.

Regulatory authority was assigned to whichever agency seemed most appropriate at the time. For some policy areas, oversight is split among several agencies—the antithesis of a systems approach.

What a mess. The USDA, historically and by law a dedicated supporter of corporate industrial food production—Big Agriculture, Big Meat, Big Dairy—is also responsible for dietary guidelines and food guides that sometimes advise the public to eat less of what these enterprises produce.

How to clean up this mess? I like to tell the story of my disheartening experience teaching a course on the farm bill, the enormous and enormously complicated legislation that governs agricultural supports and food assistance in the United States. I didn't know much about the bill when I decided to teach this course but could think of no better way to learn about it (hubris!). The high point came on the first day of class. I asked students to consider what a rational food policy might look like. They had no trouble coming up with desirable goals: make sure everyone has enough to eat at an affordable price; ensure a decent living for farmers; provide an adequate and safe livelihood for farm, restaurant, and slaughterhouse workers; protect farmers against the hazards of weather, pests, volatile markets, and climate change; produce a surplus for international trade and aid; and, most critically, promote health and protect the environment. On this last point, they thought the farm bill should encourage regional, seasonal, organic, and sustainable food production; promote conservation of soil, land, and forests; protect water and air quality, natural resources, and wildlife; and stipulate that farm animals be raised humanely.

OK, it's a long list, but policies addressing such matters already exist. They just need to be refocused on health and environmental goals, and agencies need to work together to achieve them. The difficulty of making this happen, alas, is again best illustrated by the Government Accountability Office's forty-year campaign for a single food safety agency.

In 2015, food journalists Mark Bittman and Michael Pollan, along with food policy leaders Ricardo Salvador and Olivier De Schutter, called for an overall national food policy that would directly link food production and consumption to public health and environmental protection. Given political realities, they did not recommend creation of a single agency to oversee the entire food system, but they came close. They suggested reconfiguring the USDA to become the U.S. Department of Food, Health, and Wellbeing, and appointing a National Food Policy Advisor to coordinate food policies across all government departments.

In my book *Safe Food,* I included the wildly complex organizational chart of the then-newly formed Department of Homeland Security, an entity cobbled together from about four dozen federal agencies. A single food agency would be much less complicated, but evidently less politically feasible. As for a National Food Policy Advisor? I want that job!

Running down the table, I'd make sure agricultural policies promote health and protect the environment. I'd make alcohol labels consistent with food labels, and stop booze companies from aiming their marketing at low-income and minority groups. I'd insist that environmental policies do what they are supposed to do, that federal agencies diligently track how we produce and consume food and the effects of both on our health, and that research agencies sponsor studies of how our food system can best be configured to promote regenerative (sustainable, replenishing, carbon-sequestering) agricultural practices, as well as human and animal health. I'd insist that food assistance policies make adequate, healthy diets accessible for all participants.

I would correct decades of exploitation of farm and restaurant workers who still suffer the effects of racist 1930s legislation excluding them from minimal wage requirements and protections. I'd ensure that they are compensated fairly and have safe working conditions. For those who are undocumented, I would insist on legal protections and a route to legal status.

I'd get rid of misleading health claims and obfuscating labels on food products and do for food packages what Chile and some other Latin American countries have done: put warning labels on ultraprocessed foods and ban cartoons from junk foods marketed to kids. I'd demand that food companies take safety seriously and do more to prevent foodborne illness. I would see to it that we import healthy, sustainably produced foods, and export high-quality products. Completing the list, I'd make sure that dietary guidelines and food guides promote vegetables and discourage ultraprocessed products, and say so explicitly. Above all, I would consider agriculture, health, labor, and environmental policies as a unit, and never deal with them in isolation. That's a food-systems approach in a nutshell.

Reasonable? I think so. Possible? I would dearly love to see all this as an agenda for action. Whether or not such policy goals are currently feasible, they are well worth setting. We need clear objectives for improving tomorrow's food system as a means to guide—and inspire—today's advocacy agenda.

III

THE GLOBAL POLITICS OF DIETS, HEALTH, AND THE ENVIRONMENT

13 CAN WE FEED THE WORLD WELL?

Kerry: America's industrial farmers are fond of boasting that they "feed the world" by growing massive quantities of commodity crops like corn and soy, along with meat, poultry, dairy, and eggs, all produced on a scale that our founding fathers could never have imagined. Our industrialized agricultural system is a triumph of American ingenuity, if quantity is your only yardstick for success.

But are we feeding the world *well?* A global epidemic of obesity and diet-influenced diseases is undermining the health—and shortening the lives—of billions of people. Billions more suffer from malnutrition for lack of access to safe, nutritious food.

How can we take credit for feeding the world without shouldering at least some of the blame for the fact that our factory farms are driving an unprecedented global health crisis? Is it too naïve to hope we might reinvent the way we grow food to actually nourish people, and protect the planet, instead of harming them?

Marion: I have a term for the endlessly intoned rationale for everything that's wrong with industrial food production: the Big Excuse. This says that because nine or ten billion people in the world will need to be fed by 2050, it's OK for American farmers—Big Agriculture, really—to confine animals, impoverish and endanger farm workers, ruin the effectiveness of antibiotics, poison bees and allow an "insect apocalypse," permit herbicides to contaminate organic crops, deplete underground water resources, make water in the Midwest undrinkable, and pollute the Gulf of Mexico so badly that fish can't live in it.

I recognize that food producers do not view their work this way. They believe they are doing good by producing food for a hungry world. They complain that critics like me are unfair and out of touch with the realities of farming and rural life. Perhaps, but I have personally witnessed the effects of corporate agriculture on rural America—polluted soil, water unfit to drink, and depopulation and its distressing consequences:

boarded-up stores, movie theaters, schools, and—with dire consequences—hospitals.

As a member of the Pew Commission on Industrial Farm Animal Production in the early 2000s, I also saw first-hand how we raise animals for food. The commission undertook a two-year study to research and develop recommendations for addressing the problems caused by concentrated animal feeding operations (CAFOs). To conduct the study, we visited cattle and pig CAFOs, dairy farms, chicken farms, and egg farms, some of them organic. These were the best of the lot— places where managers felt confident enough about their production practices to allow us to visit. Even so, some of these practices made us uncomfortable: laying hens in cages too small to allow wingspread, broiler chickens so crowded as to give new meaning to the term "free-range," and pungent open waste "lagoons."

And then there were the pig crates. Reading about them had not prepared me for seeing pregnant sows confined in a cage so tight that all they could do was lie down and stand up. Crating, apparently, prevents sows in crowded conditions from crushing their piglets. As an antidote, the celebrated sustainable meat producer Bill Niman, who was also on the commission, arranged for some of us to visit one of the farms producing pigs for what was then his company. There, sows wandered around in large open areas enclosed by electric fences, wallowing in mud, each housed in her own lean-to. Did they crush their piglets? Of course not. Did this method produce as many piglets per sow as industrial methods? Not quite, but the sows were treated better, the piglets thrived, and the meat was of better quality. It also was more expensive—an issue we must never forget in these discussions.

But to the question at hand: Can kinder and more sustainable methods for raising animals—and crops, for that matter—feed the world? As I see it, "feeding the world" is a convenient myth. American farmers are happy to sell surplus food to countries that can pay for it. In 2018, ten countries exported more food products to sub-Saharan Africa than did the United States.

And let's not forget that American farmers send a full 40 percent of the corn they produce to be processed into ethanol, at virtually no gain in usable energy. This bizarre feature of the U.S. food system is the result of a 2007 fuel standards law that requires billions of gallons of ethanol to be blended into automobile and jet fuels. Demands for ethanol are a strong incentive for farmers to produce even more corn, even in places where this crop should not be grown because of inadequate soil and limited rainfall. Ethanol policy is about supporting corn farmers and ethanol producers, not feeding hungry people. We don't need *more* food; we need *better* food, produced more sustainably and distributed more equitably.

We have never done a great job of getting U.S. food to international populations who need it. Years ago, a colleague and I wrote a case study about U.S. emergency food aid for Somalia. Then, food aid was often delayed, spoiled, sidetracked, or sold on the open market. It also had unintended consequences; it undermined local food production by getting people accustomed to eating imported grains. Fortunately, times have changed and the United States now joins other nations in mostly substituting cash for food donations.

If we really want the world fed adequately, we ought to be doing all we can to help populations feed themselves. This means supporting local food systems with education, particularly for women; training in sustainable farming methods; and investment in roads, transportation, and local markets. Jobs would also help, as would political stability, and, we can only hope, the absence of war and viral pandemics. It's disheartening that so much of this seems politically impossible, especially in places where leadership is corrupt and captured by corporate interests.

I see two distinctly different issues in your question: feeding the world (the myth), and reforming our agricultural system (the necessity). Separating these issues clearly exposes the external costs of industrial food production to health and the environment. Industrial agriculture is not going away in the immediate future, but we can reasonably ask whether it can be accomplished in ways that are better for the health of eaters, workers, animals, and the environment.

It can, but doing so requires action by government. Good governance is essential. The first lesson learned from my experience on that Pew commission is that Congress has already passed laws that require better production practices; it just doesn't insist that they be enforced. We could start by enforcing existing laws and then pass some new ones. We don't allow untreated human waste to be dumped into the environment, yet that's what happens with animal waste; this practice should be illegal. Polluters should pay for the damage they cause. We need laws to support more sustainable—regenerative—farming methods, welfare for food animals, better wages and working conditions for farm and slaughterhouse workers, and incentives for growing food rather than feed or fuel.

None of these improvements can happen without strong and sustained public demand—civil society in action. As members of society, we have to choose between a healthier food system and one focused on keeping food as cheap as possible. In the context of income and social inequality, promoting a healthier food system can appear elitist. Those of us willing and able to pay more for food must also do all we can to create a stronger and more thoughtful safety net for people vulnerable to the impact of higher food prices, while also addressing the political causes of this vulnerability. These actions also create economic dilemmas that are difficult to resolve in our current political era. If the world's population is to be fed adequately and healthfully in the future, everyone involved in the food system needs to be addressing these dilemmas, and right away.

14 IS THE "FREE" MARKET THE PATH TO A STABLE GLOBAL FOOD SUPPLY?

Kerry: America's capitalists love to tout our supply-and-demand-based free-market economy as an ideal economic model, the proverbial rising tide that lifts all boats. But in my view, our "free" market is about as free as "reality" shows are real.

For example, the USDA puts its thumb on the scale in favor of commodity crops at the expense of what it calls "specialty crops," those wholesome fruits and vegetables it keeps telling us we need to eat more of. Lobbyists seeking to boost the bottom lines of the agribusiness behemoths they represent are pretty much writing our ag policies.

The hidden costs of this not-so-free market system become more apparent all the time. Yet we seem determined to push our brand of agriculture on developing nations, where limited resources make it difficult to provide the secure food supply that is essential to maintain a stable society. Why do we keep doing this?

Marion: The short answer: our investment system demands ongoing growth. To please investors, Big Ag and Big Food must continuously expand—"grow"—their markets. Wall Street requires that publicly traded corporations maximize shareholder value and profits. This leaves food companies with one reason for existence: selling products. Stock prices must rise. Profits, like the universe, must ever expand.

You and I may agree with the United Nations that every man, woman, and child on Earth has the right to adequate, healthy food, but that is not how free-market capitalism works. Capitalism converts food—a substance essential for life—into a commodity to be bought and sold like any other widget.

In my experience talking about such matters, capitalism is the "C-word," never to be discussed in polite society. Americans do not like having to think about politics, let alone the power relationships that govern how food is produced, sold, and consumed. But food *is* political, very much so. Those of us who care about such matters need to recognize—and engage with—politics in order to make food systems more sustainable, less wasteful, and healthier for body and soul.

If you love food and care about how it is produced, you need to bring the C-word out of the closet, understand what capitalism does right, and deal directly with what it does wrong. Capitalism is not the only explanation for hunger, chronic disease, and environmental damage, but it is a useful starting point for understanding why such problems exist. If we want to create a food movement with real power, we need to know what we are up against.

Following the money is a useful strategy for beginning to understand basic questions elicited by our current food system. Why are so many people too poor to buy food? Why do so many impoverished people gain weight and develop chronic diseases? Why are fresh fruits and vegetables expensive in comparison to ultraprocessed junk foods? Why can't young farmers afford to buy land? Why is American agriculture aimed at producing feed for animals and fuel for cars rather than food for people? Why don't farm and restaurant workers earn decent wages? Why are slaughterhouse workers treated so badly? How did food and water—essential for our very existence—get transformed into commodities to be bought and sold for profit?

In basking in the abundance of our food system, we allowed capitalist values—free-market ideology (or, if you prefer, neoliberalism)—to dominate, regardless of the consequences. These values are easily summarized: commodify everything possible, reduce labor and production costs, maximize profits, and relentlessly oppose anyone or anything that threatens those profits. A capitalist food system keeps costs to a bare minimum, and provides an overabundance of cheap food, consequences be damned.

These consequences are also easily summarized: poor health, loss of small and medium-sized family farms, depopulation of farming communities, rural-to-urban migration, low wages and miserable working conditions for farm, slaughterhouse, and restaurant workers, ever-widening economic inequality, and increasing damage to air, soil, water, and land.

Food capitalism has always been global and continues to be. People in low-income countries are understandably tired of being poor. They want what we have and view American and European food and drink brands as symbols of status and prosperity. Food companies invest billions of marketing dollars in Africa, Asia, and Latin America to encourage such views, often at the expense of traditional local food systems. In my book *Soda Politics,* I wrote about the introduction of Coca-Cola into Myanmar, a country where sugary carbonated beverages had never been sold. If, as a result of that introduction, Myanmar's population gains weight and develops type 2 diabetes, the company takes no responsibility. Heart disease and type 2 diabetes are externalized costs of capitalism.

Another example can be observed in the effects of NAFTA (the North American Free Trade Agreement) in Mexico. That country used to be self-sufficient in food and able to export surpluses, but NAFTA required Mexico to accept imports of subsidized, overproduced, and cheaper corn from the United States. These imports undersold the corn grown by small-scale Mexican farmers, put them out of business, and forced them to abandon their land, migrate to cities, disrupt their historical food traditions, and adopt diets based on cheaper and widely advertised food products. The increase in chronic disease was predictable.

As I write this, about 10 percent of Mexican children are still observed to be undernourished, while close to 70 percent of adults are overweight or obese—right up there with the highest percentages in the world. Type 2 diabetes is rampant; it affects about 15 percent of Mexican adults and is second only to heart disease as a leading cause of death. Mexico is now a net food importer, particularly of corn and soybeans that end up in animal feed or as ingredients in ultraprocessed foods. The painful irony? Mexico largely exports healthy foods—tomatoes, peppers, avocados, and other fruits and vegetables—that are now too expensive for much of its population to afford. This too is a predictable outcome of an economic system in which profits take precedence over any other human value.

Businesses, food and otherwise, have every right to be profitable and pay dividends to investors. But couldn't we set some limits on unfettered capitalistic practices so as to encourage healthier food choices and prevent environmental damage? I'd like to think that we, as a society, could require corporations that profit from our devotion to their brands to return some of those profits in the form of better salaries, working conditions, safety practices, and product quality, as well as more sustainable supply chains.

That this is not too much to ask seems to be getting through to corporate America. In 2019, nearly two hundred members of the Business Roundtable signed a pledge to bring social values back into their missions, and the World Economic Forum restated that companies should serve all stakeholders, including society at large, by honoring diversity, improving working conditions, and respecting human rights throughout their entire supply chains.

Even if these pledges amount to no more than public relations—witness worker layoffs in response to Covid-19—they indicate that businesses, including some food companies, recognize that challenges to free-market ideology are gaining strength and must be taken seriously if companies are to continue to be profitable. Our challenge as food-system advocates is to hold food companies accountable for their promises as well as their practices. Our even bigger challenge is to change the system. How about joining the movement to get money out of politics and repeal the Supreme Court's Citizens United decision that allows corporations to buy elections. How about passing laws requiring corporations to prioritize social values and act accordingly. If we want our food system to promote health and sustainability, these kinds of changes are the ones that will count.

15 CAN WE STOP AGRICULTURE FROM CONTRIBUTING TO GLOBAL WARMING?

Kerry: Our food chain and climate change are inextricably intertwined. How we produce food, how we transport it, where we buy it, what we choose to eat, how we discard the food we don't eat; these things all play a role in altering our climate, for better or worse.

The flip side of the food/climate coin is the alarming number of ways that climate change is throwing a monkey wrench into our food chain. Farmers have always been at the mercy of nature, but this "new normal" is creating extreme weather conditions that pose unprecedented challenges: more—and more severe—droughts, floods, fires, hurricanes, and tornadoes; algae blooms and rising tides and groundwater; crop-killing pest and disease outbreaks; and other forms of environmental degradation that make it ever harder to grow the crops we depend on.

Is there any way that we can transform this vicious cycle into a virtuous loop?

Marion: I take climate change personally; I wilt in hot weather. While I was pondering your questions, July 2019 turned out to be the hottest month on record. I have two other personal measures. In November 2016, I went to Barrow, Alaska (now Utqiaġvik), as far above the Arctic Circle as you can get in the United States, to give a talk at the public library. While there, I visited the National Oceanic and Atmospheric Administration (NOAA) observatory on the outskirts of town. As a parting souvenir, its director gave me a vial of air he had just sampled for its level of carbon dioxide: 405 parts per million. Shocking. I knew that 350 was considered the upper limit of climate safety, and 400 the turning point for irreversibility. By 2020, the level exceeded 420. The last time carbon dioxide levels were that high was about three million years ago, when our oceans were fifty to eighty feet higher. Things do not look good for coastal dwellers.

I also see the effects of climate change on what I can grow in pots on my Manhattan terrace. In 1990, when I moved into the apartment in which I still live, my zip code was in the USDA's plant-hardiness zone 6b. In 2012, the USDA revised the zone maps. I haven't budged, but I now live in zone 7b, with winters expected to be an average of five degrees warmer. The upside: my rosemary plant now survives the winter, and I am taking a chance on a fig tree.

As I look at climate change, I see food systems connecting to it in two distinct ways: climate affects agriculture, but agriculture also affects climate. We can easily see what climate change is doing to agriculture. Just look at what happened in 2019. In many areas of America's heartland, farmers could not plant corn when they usually do because their fields were water-logged from snowmelt and torrential spring rains. Floods also inundated half a million acres of forest and farmland in the Mississippi Delta, and those areas remained flooded for more than six months. Farming can move northward, I suppose, as maple syrup production is already having to do, but states in the north are also hit hard by weather extremes.

It's bad enough that climate change makes planting difficult and reduces crop yields, but I am starting to see evidence that it may also reduce the nutrient content of certain crops. Researchers who grow food plants under experimental conditions of high carbon dioxide levels report alarming results: vegetables make lower levels of B-vitamins, beans make less protein, and rice makes less of both. Plants synthesize vitamins and protein on their own, but when carbon dioxide levels are high, rice also has lower levels of minerals such as zinc and iron. This could mean that the plants cannot absorb as much of these minerals from the soil.

You might think that studies like these would set off alarm bells, but not in today's political climate. Some of these studies were done by a USDA scientist who felt obliged to resign from the agency when officials questioned his findings, suppressed press coverage, and refused to allow him to discuss his work in public.

If we have passed the point of no return on carbon emissions, can we do anything to keep this situation from getting worse? For this, we need to take a look at what industrial agriculture does to climate, effects that are largely invisible to non-scientists. I collect estimates of the percentage of greenhouse gas emissions contributed by agriculture and find them highly entertaining. They range from 5 percent to 35 percent of the total, and sometimes go as high as 50 percent when they include the environmental costs of transportation, refrigeration, and agrochemical production.

I can guess who is doing the estimating from the percentage. Climate-change deniers insist on the low range; everyone else supports higher estimates. The U.S. Environmental Protection Agency says agriculture accounts for about 9 percent of American greenhouse gas emissions. But even the rather conservative World Bank says that on a global basis, agriculture is responsible for 25 percent, of which 10 percent is the result of what is happening to land and forests—the destruction of the Amazon rainforest to grow soybeans, for example. Half of the remaining 15 percent comes from beef cattle and dairy cows, thanks to "ruminant enteric fermentation" (methane burps), wastes, and manure management, and the other half from fertilizers, energy use, and methane from rice cultivation.

This last surprised me. I was not aware that rice production was so climate-unfriendly. Rice is typically grown in fields flooded to keep weeds under control, inducing bacteria to produce methane and nitrous oxide gases, both of which are much greater contributors to global warming than carbon dioxide.

These findings should encourage widespread support for regenerative agriculture, a set of practices aimed at reversing global warming by capturing and retaining carbon in soils, replenishing soil nutrients, promoting biodiversity, and conserving water. To me, regenerative practices sound a lot like the original intent of organic agriculture and what is meant by terms such as "sustainability" and "agroecology." The overall idea? Preserve soil resources and put back what you take out.

Getting government to support regenerative agriculture calls for actions that seem unimaginable in today's political environment, starting with the need for international agreements to protect forests and jungles, to plant carbon-sequestering trees everywhere possible, to reduce the number of ruminant animals, and to use other methods for growing rice—all while keeping the people who do this work safe and adequately compensated.

All of this is without considering the apparently unspeakable: the benefits to be gained from reducing population growth. Everything about this idea is fraught with politics. It doesn't help that birth control runs counter to the religious and moral beliefs of many cultures, or that attempts to control family size sometimes reduce the numbers of female children. Population control also gets into matters of us versus them: other people ought to have fewer children, but not us. This too is about politics. With rising income and greater economic, social, and gender equality, populations tend to have fewer children. Reducing inequalities seems like an especially humane way to have fewer mouths to feed.

Doing something about climate change means putting global interests above personal interests and making decisions—and sacrifices—for the good of society, something many governments seem loath to even discuss. This leaves prevention of further climate change in the hands of civil society. We can ask what it would take to mobilize civil action to the point where governments would feel forced to respond. In 2019, demonstrations demanding government action on climate change took place in eighty countries, largely led by young people who recognize that they face a future of increasing desertification, catastrophic weather, food shortages, and, in consequence, massive migration and conflict. I have no doubt that these demonstrations will have an impact eventually, but sooner would be better than later.

We Americans cannot take the moral high road on this issue when our own government refuses to join international climate-change agreements. Climate change is a global problem. People everywhere must join together to deal with it. If only there were an easy way to make that happen.

16 WILL TECHNOLOGY FIX OUR FOOD SYSTEM?

⌐━━━━

Kerry: "Agropreneurs" are pouring enormous resources into creating a more resilient food chain. Robots that can harvest fruits and vegetables? Inevitable, just like self-driving cars. Pollinator drones? Already being tested in fruit and nut orchards from California to New York.

I asked you earlier about lab-grown meats. This "cellular agriculture" now even includes bugs. Tufts University recently published a paper with the unappetizing title "Possibilities for Engineered Insect Tissue as a Food Source."

Indoor vertical farms have been on the rise for years, but for sheer novelty you can't beat Rotterdam's floating dairy farm. Designed to withstand hurricanes, it houses roughly forty cows, along with manure-cleaning and milking robots. While this sounds wildly unnatural, what's natural about the way we do industrial dairy now?

Is it me, or is there a distinctly dystopian flavor to all of these enterprises?

Marion: A technology-driven food system? What leaps to my mind is Soylent, the liquid meal replacement named ironically (I hope) for the dystopian 1973 film *Soylent Green*. In this film's terrifying vision, unchecked population growth and environmental degradation have created a situation so desperate that only the very rich have access to fresh food and clean water. Everyone else subsists on Soylent Green, wafers reconstituted from—spoiler alert—human bodies: "Soylent is people!" This nightmare may be extreme, but the conditions leading up to it are with us right now.

Technologically challenged foodie that I am, I don't have much interest in the wonders of modern food technology—what I call techno-foods. As I've mentioned, one of my personal food rules is to avoid eating foods with artificial ingredients that humans did not evolve to consume. But because investors are pouring tons of money into techno-foods, and many people like these products (witness plant-based meat substitutes), I try to keep an open mind about them.

To that end, I accept every invitation I can to visit or give talks at food-tech shows. These are fun. I love watching machines make 3-D cookies and pizza. Other exhibitors have loftier goals—growing salad greens indoors, for example. I was dubious about this too, especially after noting the bland taste of some grown hydroponically in a truck. These, I was told, were designed to meet the specifications of the chefs who were buying them (remind me not to go to their restaurants).

But then I visited the AeroFarms factory in New Jersey. In a space the size of an airplane hangar, this company is growing tiny greens on brightly lit floor-to-ceiling racks. I had some doubts about AeroFarms' claims that it takes "indoor vertical farming to a new level of precision and productivity with minimal environmental impact and virtually zero risk." The precision and productivity were obvious. The company measures the nutrient levels of its greens, and theirs had amounts as good or better than those of conventionally grown products. Environmental impact is relative, however, and this factory uses masses of electricity rather than energy derived from the sun.

When I tasted the greens, I knew I had to take this method seriously. Their flavors were distinct, bright, and fresh. This factory sells what it produces at a price equivalent to that of its competitors, and its greens get to local stores quickly. As I learned when doing the research for *What to Eat,* it can take two weeks for vegetables grown in California to get to my local New York City supermarket. On the basis of taste and freshness, AeroFarms' greens are a better option. I remain skeptical—that's my job, after all—but a bit less so with respect to indoor farming.

My more important question about the role of food technology is what it can do to address health and environmental problems related to food systems. I have been following the plans for technological solutions to global warming—reflecting sunlight back into space, sucking carbon dioxide out of the atmosphere, or bioengineering *E. coli* to subsist on carbon dioxide— but we are far from knowing how to do any of this on a large enough scale to assess whether these methods might work, let alone worry about their unintended consequences.

Hunger, chronic disease, and global warming are not technological problems; they are social, economic, and political problems requiring social, economic, and political solutions. Their causes are rooted in how our societies function and in the lack of political will to address these problems in any meaningful way. Focusing on technological approaches, no matter how entertaining or potentially useful, distracts us from engaging food corporations, governments, and civil society in addressing these problems right now. The concentration of resources on the distantly beneficial technology sector also shifts investment away from regenerative agriculture and smaller scale farming, which could sequester carbon immediately.

Consider genetically modified foods (GMOs). In 1994, the strongest moral argument for inducing the FDA to approve this technology was that GMOs would increase food production and eliminate hunger. GMO crops, their makers said, could be bioengineered to withstand conditions of harsh climate, poor soil, and limited water in low-income countries. Today, GMO corn and soy dominate industrial agriculture everywhere they are grown, but they are used mainly to feed animals, fuel cars, and produce profits for Big Agriculture. They are not doing much to feed people with limited resources.

I see two reasons for the failure of GMO technology

to address world food needs. The first is the money: small farmers in low-income countries cannot afford to pay enough for GMO seeds to make it worthwhile for biotechnology companies to invest in the kind of research these farmers need. The second is the science: the technical problems involved in such research are formidable.

In my book *Safe Food,* I wrote about Golden Rice, the poster child for the benefits of food biotechnology. This rice is bioengineered to contain high levels of beta-carotene, a precursor of vitamin A; a deficiency of this vitamin is a major cause of blindness in low-income countries. The idea behind Golden Rice is to put beta-carotene into a food that everyone eats. In theory, this makes sense. But in practice? *Safe Food* lists the steps required to engineer, grow, and get this rice to market. The book first appeared in 2003, but by 2020 this rice was still unavailable for consumption, mostly because of technical problems that arose during its bioengineering and field production.

Golden Rice may yet prove beneficial, but here too I remain skeptical. In areas of widespread vitamin A deficiency, fruits and vegetables rich in beta-carotene are easy to grow. But people may not have the means to grow or buy them, may avoid eating them for cultural reasons, or are so burdened with intestinal worms that they cannot absorb beta-carotene. These barriers call for cultural, social, economic—and health—interventions.

We don't need technology to make sure everyone has enough money for food, to create a healthier food supply, or to encourage food production and consumption practices that are healthier, more sustainable, and less wasteful. If we view technology as the answer to food-system problems, I fear that the future really will be dystopian. Yes, technology has its uses. But if it is utopia we want, we will have to advocate for it. We will have to oppose unhealthful and unsustainable corporate practices and insist that governments do everything they can—and they can do a lot—to create food systems as much or more for people as for profit. We need a systems fix, not a techno-fix.

17 WHAT ARE SUSTAINABLE DEVELOPMENT GOALS, AND WHY SHOULD WE CARE?

Kerry: You introduced me to the concept of Sustainable Development Goals (SDGs), an international initiative which I don't hear about much here in the United States. This must surely be a disappointment to the United Nations General Assembly, which in 2015 created seventeen goals to address global problems, among them eliminating poverty and hunger, reducing inequality, promoting good health, advocating responsible consumption, and supporting peace, justice, decent work, and economic growth. The intent of the SDGs is to achieve these goals by the year 2030.

Do you think the SDGs have the potential to have any meaningful impact on our food systems? Can you imagine Americans ever embracing this epic global agenda?

Marion: Epic, indeed. When I give public lectures, I like to wear one of the SDG pins I've acquired: a circle of the colors standing for each of the goals, a similar circle with the logo of the UN's Food and Agriculture Organization (FAO), a square that says Zero Hunger, and another with its Spanish translation—#HambreCero. The last two state SDG goal 2, which the FAO adopted as its primary focus for action. I wear these pins out of respect and admiration for the enormous effort undertaken by UN agencies to set measurable targets for sustainable development and to hold countries accountable for achieving them. Buried among these targets are several aimed at solving problems caused by dysfunctional food systems.

I can understand why hardly anyone in the United States has heard of the SDGs. For one thing, there are too many—seventeen goals, each with its own set of sub-goals. For another, they exist at the level of government policy, which all too often affects daily lives in ways we don't easily recognize.

The SDGs remind me of the U.S. Healthy People initiative, which I know about because in the late 1980s I worked in the government office that developed them. This initiative began in the 1970s and continues today.

Like the SDGs, it is an enormous effort involving enormous numbers of government and private-sector organizations. Unlike the SDGs, Healthy People focuses exclusively on health issues, for which it sets specific and measurable ten-year objectives. One of the 2020 objectives, for example, is to reduce the prevalence of food insecurity and hunger among Americans from 14.6 percent in 2008 to 6.0 percent in 2030. The goal is laudable, but the Healthy People process does not say who is responsible for achieving it or how it is to be achieved.

A similar lack of who and how affects the SDGs. They do indeed cover a lot of territory. None of them mentions food or food systems in its title, although Zero Hunger comes closest; its sub-heading states, "Achieve food security and improved nutrition and promote sustainable agriculture." You have to search through the sub-goals to see that food and nutrition are embedded in or implied by practically all of them. Sub-goal 12.3, as I mentioned in chapter 11, is to cut food waste by half.

The SDGs have some noticeable gaps. They have little to say about reducing the consequences of obesity, for example. It takes some digging to discover that sub-goal 2.2 ("By 2030, end all forms of malnutrition") comes with indicator 2.2.2, which calls for measuring the prevalence of malnutrition—both wasting and overweight—among children under age five. But obesity affects nearly two billion people, adults as well as children, and is a major risk factor for type 2 diabetes, coronary heart disease, and other conditions that the development community collectively refers to as noncommunicable diseases (NCDs). These come up only in sub-goal 3.4: "By 2030, reduce by one-third premature mortality from noncommunicable diseases through prevention and treatment and promote mental health and well-being."

It also takes work to figure out where food and nutrition fit into the SDGs. Nutritionists argue that nutrition is integral to every one of the seventeen goals in some way, since people cannot function if they are not adequately nourished, but I think the absence of more explicit statements is an unfortunate omission.

Searching is also needed to find the widely scattered sub-goals for improving food systems. Sub-goal 6.1 calls for universal and equitable access to safe and affordable drinking water by 2030. Sub-goal 14.4 deals with fishing, but more urgently; it calls for regulating harvesting and ending overfishing by 2020. Sub-goal 15.2 is about improving land use—implementing sustainable forest management, halting deforestation, and restoring degraded forests by 2020, a particularly demanding priority given the widespread burning of the Amazon rainforest in 2019 and 2020.

UN agencies necessarily operate through leadership and consensus among 193 member nations and have no real power to require state action. But in agreeing to the SDGs, nations also agreed to conduct regular progress reviews. The UN publishes annual reports based on information provided by its members, and its 2018 report highlighted heartening reductions in maternal and childhood mortality and noted that more than a hundred countries have introduced initiatives for sustainable food production and consumption.

But most goals show little chance of achievement. The most discouraging measures are those demonstrating the increase in global temperatures and the lack of progress in achieving Zero Hunger. World hunger is on the rise again, and stunting, wasting, and overweight still affect millions of children under age five, especially those in low-income families. The lack of progress toward the SDGs make it clear that when goals are politically inconvenient, governments conveniently ignore them.

So why should anyone care about the SDGs, or the Healthy People initiative for that matter? I can think of three reasons. First, governments and organizations in many countries use them to set agendas for action and advocacy. Second, without them, it is impossible to measure progress or hold governments accountable. Third, the SDGs have inspired nongovernmental organizations (NGOs) in civil society to take up one or another goal as their particular cause for action. Ironically, food companies have done so too. I particularly treasure a graphic claiming that "Monsanto's work contributes to all 17 SDGs" (it does not say how).

I suspect that part of the reason for eager adoption and use of the SDGs is their gorgeously designed, brightly colored graphics and instantly recognizable symbols (hence, my pins). The UN cannot force governments to act, but it can inspire them—and civil society organizations—to do so.

The UN also aims to inspire individual engagement. It issued a "Lazy person's guide to saving the world." This lists climate-friendly things we can do at home (eat less meat, poultry, and fish), outside the home (don't buy more food than we need; shop for sustainable seafood), and at work (don't waste food; recycle). Even more strongly, the guide encourages us to get involved in politics, particularly as related to climate change: "Speak up! Ask your company and Government to engage in initiatives that will not harm people or the planet. Voice your support for Paris [climate change] Agreement!" Those of us who care about food-system issues can use the SDGs to direct our own advocacy for reducing hunger, the health effects of obesity, and climate change.

18 IS THERE A ROAD MAP TO THE FUTURE OF FOOD?

Kerry: Agriculture is said to be the origin of civilization. When humans learned to cultivate crops, we made the transition from a nomadic hunter-gatherer way of life to putting down roots in one place. This seismic shift led to the creation of stable communities with a relatively secure food supply.

Ironically, our current agricultural practices are arguably *destabilizing* civilization by fostering disease, worsening climate change, threatening the world's ability to grow food, and leaving large numbers of people unable to pay for healthy diets.

It feels as if we're heading for a global meltdown. Are we? And, if we are, what can any one person do about it? What *is* anyone doing about it? We have a food movement, but is it doing anything to fix the inequities in our food system?

Marion: We are not *headed* for a global meltdown; we are in one. Look at Greenland's melting glaciers. On August 1, 2019, they poured a record-breaking 12.5 *billion* tons of water into the Atlantic Ocean. But what you are asking gets right to the most critical dilemma: Can the world's growing population be fed decently without further heating up the climate and making even more people hungry and chronically ill?

This is precisely the question addressed by two groups of international experts commissioned by *The Lancet,* which published their reports ten days apart in January 2019. The first is called EAT-Lancet, after its EAT Forum sponsor, a nonprofit group devoted to food-system transformation. The EAT-Lancet Commission reviewed evidence linking current diets to damage to health and the environment. On that basis, it developed the Planetary Health Diet, which calls on people in resource-rich countries to cut current meat consumption by half but to double their intake of vegetables, fruits, and nuts.

As you might imagine, the meat industry reacted strongly to this. But EAT-Lancet's proposed diet also induced criticism on other grounds: its unrealistic specificity (no more than 28 grams of meat, 31 grams of sugar, or 50 grams of potatoes a day, for example), its seemingly vegetarian agenda, the alleged hypocrisy and conflicted interests of the founders of the EAT Forum, the inappropriateness of the recommended diet for low-income countries, and its high cost.

The cost complaint merits comment. For reasons of policy and politics, the prices of healthier foods tend to be higher than those of ultraprocessed foods. Food costs amount to only a small percentage of the income of people with money; the U.S. average is less than 10 percent. But an investigation of the price of more than 700 foods in 159 countries came to a sobering conclusion: the Planetary Health Diet is so expensive that its cost would exceed the incomes of more than 1.5 billion people, many of them in sub-Saharan Africa and South Asia.

But the other criticisms, and their vehemence, surprised me. I thought they must be coming from people who had not read the report carefully, if at all—perhaps understandably, given its fifty pages of small print and dense writing. The EAT-Lancet Commission provided illustrations of meals consistent with the Planetary

Health Diet. To me, these looked much like the meals illustrating the USDA's MyPlate food guide in 2011, with fruits and vegetables on half the plate and grains on another quarter. Except for the gram-level specificity of the proposed diet and its updated research review, I did not think the EAT-Lancet report offered much that was new. But much of the reaction to it demonstrated how unrealistic—and, therefore, insensitive—dietary advice for resource-rich populations can appear to people in low- and middle-income countries, as well as to poor and less privileged people in countries like the United States.

In contrast, I viewed the report from the second Lancet Commission, "The Global Syndemic of Obesity, Undernutrition, and Climate Change," as groundbreaking. Perhaps because of its obfuscating title, or its publication in the wake of the uproar over the previous week's EAT-Lancet report, this one received almost no press attention in the United States. This was unfortunate; the Global Syndemic report deserves to be read by everyone who cares about food-system issues. Its authors presented the clearest road map I have seen to address the Big Three food-system problems—hunger, noncommunicable diseases, climate change—at one and the same time (hence "syndemic," a term derived from medical anthropology meaning multiple, concurrent, and interrelated epidemics).

This report's great strength is its hard-headed identification of the source of these problems in "consumptogenic" economic systems, the euphemism it uses for capitalism. Such systems enable food corporations to hold power, public goods to be privatized, companies to externalize the costs of production, and governments to be so thoroughly captured that they fail to address the risks of corporate power. It identifies the barriers—collectively, policy inertia—to fixing these problems: strong food industry opposition in the presence of weak governance and weak civil society.

What to do? The report calls for four "triple-duty" actions to simultaneously address hunger, obesity, and climate change: eat less red meat, issue sustainable dietary guidelines, regulate the food industry, and establish a policy framework that deals with food systems as a whole.

Regulate the food industry? This is the first time I have ever seen that suggestion in a major international report. The Global Syndemic report gives explicit guidelines for such action: end subsidies and tax breaks for food corporations, require companies to pay the externalized costs of what they produce, block them from fighting public health measures, keep them out of public policy decisions, require them to disclose conflicts of interests and political donations, and hold them fully accountable for the damage they cause to health and the environment—and to democratic institutions.

This looks to me like an agenda for advocacy. In this day and age, replacing capitalism with an economic system that promotes planetary health may seem inconceivably unrealistic, but reforming the current system does not. If we cannot get governments to regulate corporations, we had best turn our attention to strengthening civil society, meaning organized groups (NGOs) and grassroots advocates willing to join in common cause.

Public pressures have already forced some food companies to issue statements about social values, reformulate their products, and reduce the waste they generate. It may be hard for those of us immersed in the day-to-day work of addressing the food problems that most concern us—school food, farmers' markets, food insecurity, fair trade, food labels, waste—to pay attention to global needs for food-system change, but it's worth trying to see the bigger picture. If we want better food systems, we need to have a clear idea of what we want changed and how to make that change happen. For that, we need to become effective advocates.

How? As I have said or implied all along, the questions of how to get involved in advocacy and how best to achieve advocacy goals deserve their own discussion. Read on.

CONCLUSION

Take Action

Throughout this book, I've called for advocacy for a healthier and more sustainable food system. In the United States alone, hundreds of advocacy groups are working on these issues. Collectively, they constitute a food movement, although one fragmented among groups with widely disparate and separate goals: health, the environment, agricultural sustainability, workers' rights, animal welfare, food security, and everything else I've talked about in this book. These range from the personal (better diets) to the political (improved food environments).

Advocating for any of these goals is a step in the right direction. Promoting better dietary choices improves individual health, but it also supports the farmers, producers, and food service operations promoting food-system change. Voting with forks sets an example

and encourages others to care about how food is produced, sold, and marketed, by whom, and under what
conditions. We can argue about whether advocacy for
better personal diets constitutes a movement or is just
a secular trend, but "Good Food" advocacy has already
forced food companies to reformulate products, clean
up their supply chains, and publicly recognize demands
for more responsible corporate behavior.

I give the Good Food movement credit for improving the quality of fresh foods in supermarkets, the
increased availability of farmers' markets and organic
foods, greater public interest in food issues, and my
personal favorite, the increasing presence of food studies programs at universities. When my NYU department
initiated foods studies programs in 1996, these were
unique; now many colleges offer such opportunities.

Those of us who vote with our forks have the means
to do so. But what about people who do not? Organic
foods are expensive. Fruits and vegetables are expensive. Cooking requires skills, equipment, and time.
Not everyone can afford a university program in food
studies. Arguing for better dietary choices can easily
appear elitist, insensitive to cultural, racial, gender, and

economic disparities, and out of touch with the reality of people's daily lives.

I hear such charges all the time. I take them seriously, and so do most food advocates I know. They must be addressed, not least because they get right to the point I most want to emphasize. For real and lasting improvements in the food system, we must do more than vote with forks. We must vote with votes, engage in politics, and advocate for food systems that distribute benefits not just to corporations, but also to people who need and deserve those benefits. This means creating a food environment in which the healthy and sustainable food choice becomes the easy choice—more readily available, affordable, and acceptable.

How to start? I see nothing wrong with beginning with the low-hanging fruit: improving the food distributed in schools, food assistance programs, workplaces, hospitals, and other institutions in our hometowns, and reducing food waste. Improvements to the food environment are more challenging but not impossible. Soda tax advocacy has proved successful in many places. So have warning labels on ultraprocessed foods, restrictions on the marketing of junk food to children, and promotion of safe public water fountains. These can improve people's lives. All are easier to accomplish than systems change.

But in the long run, advocacy must address the root causes of current food-system problems. If we are to redress system inequities, we must advocate for jobs with adequate wages, education, health care, policies promoting sustainable agriculture, public transportation, and, yes, healthy food for everyone. This means advocating for government and private sector promotion of social goals, which in turn means getting corporate money out of politics, repealing the Supreme Court's Citizens United decision, and initiating public funding of election campaigns.

How do we get there from here? Methods for producing social change are well established. Individuals can make a difference, but advocacy works better when carried out by groups—the larger, more diverse, and more community based, the better. Advocacy involves community organizing or, as is taught in public health schools, program planning.

If you want to advocate, you need to work with community groups to identify the problems *they* want solved and how *they* want to solve them. Together, you research the problem, set goals for addressing it, recruit allies, identify who has the power to make the change you want, decide on strategies and tactics, and develop a campaign. Advocacy means convincing as many people as possible to join the campaign (that's where community organizing becomes critical) and using the political system to achieve goals. You and your allies do the research, write letters and position papers, and meet with legislators. If this sounds like lobbying, it is.

Students tell me that this kind of politics feels dirty to them—corrupt and corrupting. But when I was a student in the 1960s, we believed that that advocacy could change the world. We could see how our protests helped end the war in Vietnam and obtain civil rights for African Americans and women. Yes, we were naïve about the ferocity and power of the pushback, but the gains were real and many of them have lasted.

Today, advocacy still works when it is done well, meaning that it recruits the community to the cause. The Berkeley soda tax campaign is a clear example. Its organizers represented all sectors of the community. They did advocacy by the book. They worked with other community members to decide on a ballot initiative and how to conduct the campaign. They went door to door in every Berkeley neighborhood, from the low-income flats to the high-income hills, to explain the links between soda company marketing, sugary beverages, and type 2 diabetes. To the complaint that soda taxes are regressive, they had a compelling response: type 2 diabetes is regressive. This level of community involvement—along with promises, since fulfilled, that low-income residents would have a say in how the revenues would be used—led an overwhelming 76 percent of voters to favor the tax.

If you want to become a food advocate, pick the problem you want to address, find a group working on that issue, and join it. An online search will locate food advocacy groups in your area (the sources listed at the back of this book cite advocacy resources and links to lists of organizations).

Advocates face an often discouraging barrier: how to get paid for this work. Advocates are Davids up against Goliaths who have far greater resources and are rewarded handsomely for their lobbying. Another barrier is splintering: many groups working on many different issues and competing for the same funding sources. I wish I could wave a magic wand and instantly unite food advocacy organizations into huge coalitions with real power to effect change. I wish these groups would put more effort into teaching members how to become better community organizers and coalition builders, and that funders would encourage such efforts and put real money into supporting advocacy work. I wish every food movement group would devote substantial effort to lobbying for fundamental system changes as well as for its particular goal.

But even when they don't fulfill these wishes, food movement organizations are worth participation and support. They offer hope that changing the food system is possible. What else can you do as an individual? My immediate answer: run for office!

If getting that involved in politics is too much to contemplate, you still have plenty of ways to participate. Support political candidates. Volunteer for campaigns. Above all, vote. Encourage your friends and colleagues to vote. In joining the food movement, you will be doing much good for yourself, your family, your neighbors, and the world. In working to create truly equitable food systems, you also will be doing your part to preserve, promote, and sustain democracy.

ABBREVIATIONS

CAFOs	concentrated animal feeding operations
CDC	Centers for Disease Control and Prevention (of HHS)
EPA	Environmental Protection Agency
FAO	Food and Agriculture Organization (of the United Nations)
FDA	Food and Drug Administration (of HHS)
FTC	Federal Trade Commission
GAO	Government Accountability Office
HHS	U.S. Department of Health and Human Services
NASA	National Aeronautics and Space Agency
NCDs	noncommunicable diseases
NGOs	nongovernmental organizations
NIH	National Institutes of Health (of HHS)
NIMBY	Not in My Backyard

NOAA	National Oceanic and Atmospheric Administration
OSHA	Occupational Safety and Health Administration
SDGs	Sustainable Development Goals (of the United Nations)
SNA	School Nutrition Association
TTB	Alcohol and Tobacco Tax and Trade Bureau (of the Treasury Department)
USDA	U.S. Department of Agriculture
WHO	World Health Organization (of the United Nations)

SOURCES AND FURTHER READING

Note: URLs are only provided for online references that cannot be found easily by searching for their titles.

Introduction

International Panel of Experts on Sustainable Food Systems. COVID-19 and the crisis in food systems: symptoms, causes, and potential solutions. IPES-Food, April 2020.

Nestle M. A food lover's love of nutrition science, policy, and politics. *European Journal of Clinical Nutrition.* 2019;73:1551–1555.

1. What is a healthy diet?

Bowen S, Brenton J, Elliott S. *Pressure Cooker: Why Home Cooking Won't Solve Our Problems and What We Can Do About It.* New York: Oxford University Press; 2019.

FAO. Food-based dietary guidelines. Rome, 2019.

FAO, WHO. Sustainable healthy diets—guiding principles. Rome, 2019.

Lawrence MA. Ultra-processed food and adverse health outcomes. *BMJ.* 2019;365:l2289.

Monteiro CA, Cannon G, Levy RB, Moubarac J-C, Louzada MLC, Rauber F, et al. Ultra-processed foods: what they are and how to identify them. *Public Health Nutrition.* 2019;22(5):936–941.

Nestle M. Mediterranean diets: historical and research overview. *American Journal of Clinical Nutrition.* 1995;61(suppl):1313s–1320s.

———. *What to Eat.* New York: North Point Press / Farrar, Straus and Giroux; 2006.

Pollan M. *Food Rules: An Eater's Manual.* New York: Penguin; 2009.

USDA, HHS. Dietary guidelines for Americans, 2015–2020.

Willett W, Rockström J, Loken B, Springmann M, Lang T, Vermeulen S, et al. Food in the Anthropocene: the EAT-Lancet Commission on healthy diets from sustainable food systems. *Lancet.* 2019;393(10170):447–492.

2. Why does nutrition advice always seem to be changing?

Barnard ND, Long MB, Ferguson JM, Flores R, Kahleova H. Industry funding and cholesterol research: a systematic review. *American Journal of Lifestyle Medicine.* Published online December 11, 2019.

Nestle M. *Food Politics: How the Food Industry Influences Nutrition and Health.* Berkeley: University of California Press; 2002. 10th anniversary ed.; 2013. See "Appendix: Issues in Nutrition and Nutrition Research," 413–423.

——. *Unsavory Truth: How Food Companies Skew the Science of What We Eat.* New York: Basic Books; 2018.

——. *What to Eat.* New York: North Point Press / Farrar, Straus and Giroux; 2006.

USDA, HHS. Dietary guidelines for Americans, 2015–2020.

3. Are low-carb diets really better for us?

Katz DI, Meller S. Can we say what diet is best for health? *Annual Review of Public Health.* 2014;35:83–103.

Nestle M. *What to Eat.* New York: North Point Press / Farrar, Straus and Giroux; 2006.

Shan Z, Guo Y, Hu FB, Liu L, Qi Q. Association of low-carbohydrate and low-fat diets with mortality among U.S. adults. *JAMA Internal Medicine.* January 21, 2020 (epub ahead of print).

4. Can food be addictive?

Brownell KD, Gold MS. *Food and Addiction: A Comprehensive Handbook.* New York: Oxford University Press; 2012.

Hall KD, Ayuketah A, Bernstein S, Brychta R, Cai H, Cassimatis T, et al. Ultra-processed diets cause excess calorie intake and weight gain: a one-month inpatient randomized controlled trial of ad libitum food intake. *Cell Metabolism*. 2019;30(1):67–77.e3.

Moss M. *Salt Sugar Fat: How the Food Giants Hooked Us.* New York: Random House; 2013.

5. Is fake meat better for us—and the planet than the real thing?

Hu FB, Otis BO, McCarthy G. Can plant-based meat alternatives be part of a healthy and sustainable diet? *JAMA*. August 26, 2019 (epub ahead of print).

Pew Commission on Industrial Farm Animal Production. Putting meat on the table: industrial farm animal production in America. Pew Charitable Trusts and Johns Hopkins Bloomberg School of Public Health, 2008.

Specht L. Is the future of meat animal-free? *Food Technology*. 2018;72(1):16–21.

Van der Weele C, Feindt P, van der Goot AJ, van Mierlo B, van Boekel M. Meat alternatives: an integrative comparison. *Trends in Food Science and Technology*. 2019;88:505–512.

Wurgaft BA. *Meat Planet: Artificial Flesh and the Future of Food.* Oakland: University of California Press; 2019.

6. Is it a good idea to self-medicate with supplements or superfoods?

Berkeley Wellness Letter. Dietary supplements: we can do better. University of California, July 31, 2019.

Cohen PA. The supplement paradox: negligible benefits, robust consumption. *JAMA*. 2016;316(14):1453–1454.

FDA. Dietary supplements.

——. Label claims for foods and dietary supplements.

Nestle M. *Unsavory Truth: How Food Companies Skew the Science of What We Eat.* New York: Basic Books; 2018.

————. *What to Eat.* New York: North Point Press / Farrar, Straus and Giroux; 2006.

Pomeranz JL, Adler S. Defining commercial speech in the context of food marketing. *Journal of Law, Medicine and Ethics.* 2015;43(suppl 1):40–43.

Scrinis G. *Nutritionism: The Science and Politics of Dietary Advice.* New York: Columbia University Press; 2013.

7. Why should anyone go hungry, ever?

Fisher A. *Big Hunger: The Unholy Alliance between Corporate America and Anti-Hunger Groups.* Cambridge, MA: MIT Press; 2017.

Keith-Jennngs B, Llobrera J, Dean S. Links of the Supplemental Nutrition Assistance Program with food insecurity, poverty, and health: evidence and potential. *American Journal of Public Health.* 2019;109(12):1636–1640.

Nestle M. Hunger in America: a matter of policy. *Social Research.* 1999;66(1): 257–282.

————. The Supplemental Nutrition Assistance Program (SNAP): history, politics, and public health implications. *American Journal of Public Health.* 2019;109(12):1631–1635.

Nestle M, Guttmacher S. Hunger in the United States: rationale, methods, and policy implications of state hunger surveys. *Journal of Nutrition Education.* 1992;24:18s–22s.

Poppendieck J. *Breadlines Knee-Deep in Wheat: Food Assistance in the Great Depression.* Berkeley: University of California Press; 2014.

————. *Sweet Charity? Emergency Food and the End of Entitlement.* New York: Viking; 1998.

Schwartz M, Levi R, Lott M, Arm K, Seligman H. Healthy Eating Research nutrition guidelines for the charitable food system. Durham, NC: Healthy Eating Research; 2020.

Quigley WP. Five hundred years of English Poor Laws, 1349–1834: regulating the working and nonworking poor. *Akron Law Review.* 1997;30(1).

8. Is obesity really only a matter of personal responsibility?

Brownell KD. *Food Fight: The Inside Story of America's Obesity Crisis—and What We Can Do About It.* New York: McGraw-Hill; 2003.

Harris JL, Frazier W III, Kumanyika S, Ramierez AG. Rudd report: increasing disparities in unhealthy food advertising targeted to Hispanic and Black youth. Rudd Center for Food Policy and Obesity and Council on Black Health, University of Connecticut, January 2019.

Nestle M, Jacobson MF. Halting the obesity epidemic: a public health policy approach. *Public Health Reports.* 2000;115:12–24.

Nestle M, Nesheim M. *Why Calories Count: From Science to Politics.* Berkeley: University of California Press; 2012.

Young LR, Nestle M. Reducing portion sizes to prevent obesity: a call to action. *American Journal of Preventive Medicine* 2012;43(5):565–568.

9. Why isn't healthy school food a no-brainer?

Isoldi KK, Dalton S, Rodriguez DP, Nestle M. Classroom "cupcake" celebrations: observations of foods offered and consumed. *Journal of Nutrition Education and Behavior.* 2012;44(1):71–75.

Kogan R. Rollback of nutrition standards not supported by evidence. *Health Affairs.* March 13, 2019.

Nestle M. *Food Politics: How the Food Industry Influences Nutrition and Health.* Berkeley: University of California Press; 2002. 10th anniversary ed.; 2013.

———. *Soda Politics: Taking on Big Soda (and Winning).* New York: Oxford University Press; 2015.

Poppendieck J. *Free for All: Fixing School Food in America.* Berkeley: University of California Press; 2010.

Siegel BE. *Kid Food: The Challenge of Feeding Children in a Highly Processed World.* New York: Oxford University Press; 2019.

Waters A. *Edible Schoolyard: A Universal Idea.* San Francisco: Chronicle Books; 2008.

White House Task Force on Childhood Obesity. Report to the president: solving the problem of childhood obesity within a generation. The White House, May 2010.

10. Why don't we demand a higher standard of food safety?

Capel PD, McCarthy KA, Coupe RH, Grey KM, Amenumey SE, Baker NT, et al. Agriculture—a river runs through it—the connections between agriculture and water quality. U.S. Geological Survey Circular 1433, 2018.

FDA. 2018 summary report on antimicrobials sold or distributed for use in food-producing animals. December 2019.

GAO. High-risk series: substantial efforts needed to achieve greater progress on high-risk areas. GAO-19-157SP. March 2019:195–197.

Hanna-Attisha M. *What the Eyes Don't See: A Story of Crisis, Resistance, and Hope in an American City.* New York: One World; 2018.

Marler B. 10 things food safety expert, Bill Marler, does not eat. Marler Blog, June 19, 2018.

Nestle M. *Safe Food: The Politics of Food Safety.* Berkeley: University of California Press; 2003. Rev. ed.; 2013.

Rather IA, Koh WY, Paek WK, Lim J. The sources of chemical contaminants in food and their health implications. *Frontiers in Pharmacology.* 2017;8:830. Published online November 17, 2017.

Richtel M. Tainted pork, ill consumers and an investigation thwarted. *New York Times,* August 4, 2019.

11. Why can't we stop wasting food?

Flanagan K, Robertson K, Hanson C. Reducing food loss and waste: setting a global action agenda. World Resources Institute, August 2019.

GAO. Food loss and waste: building on existing federal efforts could help to achieve national reduction goal. GAO-19-391. June 2019.

USDA Economic Research Service. Food loss: estimates of food loss at the retail and consumer levels. www.ers.usda.gov/data-products/food-availability-per-capita-data-system/food-loss/

12. Do we need a national food policy agency?

Bittman M, Pollan M, Salvador R, De Schutter O. A national food policy for the 21st century. Medium.com, October 6, 2015.

Nestle M. The farm bill drove me insane. *Politico*, March 17, 2016.

Nestle M, Lee PR, Baron RB. Nutrition policy update. In: Weininger J, Briggs GM, eds. *Nutrition Update,* Vol. 1. New York: John Wiley; 1983:285–313.

Shannon KI, Kim BF, McKenzie SF, Lawrence RS. Food system policy, public health, and human rights in the United States. *Annual Review of Public Health.* 2015;356:151–173.

13. Can we feed the world well?

Congressional Research Service. U.S. international food assistance: an overview. December 6, 2018.

Leahy S. Insect "apocalypse" in U.S. driven by 50x increase in toxic pesticides. *National Geographic,* August 6, 2019.

Nestle M, Dalton S. Food aid and international hunger crises: the United States in Somalia. *Agriculture and Human Values.* 1994;11(4):19–27.

Pew Commission on Industrial Farm Animal Production. Putting meat on the table: industrial farm animal production in America. Pew Charitable Trusts and Johns Hopkins Bloomberg School of Public Health, 2008.

Schechinger AW, Cox C. Feeding the world: think U.S. agriculture will end world hunger? Think again. Environmental Working Group, October 2016.

World Integrated Trade Solution. Sub-Saharan Africa food products imports by country 2018.

14. Is the "free" market the path to a stable global food supply?

Business Roundtable. Statement on the purpose of a corporation. August 2019.

Gálvez A. *Eating NAFTA: Trade, Food Policies, and the Destruction of Mexico.* Oakland: University of California Press; 2018.

Goodman PS. Big Business pledged gentler capitalism. It's not happening in a pandemic. *New York Times,* April 13, 2020.

Holt-Giménez E. *A Foodie's Guide to Capitalism: Understanding the Political Economy of What We Eat.* New York: Monthly Review Press; 2017.

Nestle M. *Soda Politics: Taking on Big Soda (and Winning).* New York: Oxford University Press; 2015.

Otero G. *The Neoliberal Diet: Healthy Profits, Unhealthy People.* Austin: University of Texas Press; 2018.

Planet Fat. *New York Times,* May 2, 2017–January 9, 2019.

Schwab K. Davos Manifesto 2020: The universal purpose of a company in the fourth industrial revolution. World Economic Forum. December 2, 2019.

15. Can we stop agriculture from contributing to global warming?

EPA. Inventory of U.S. greenhouse gas emissions and sinks. See Draft Inventory, 1990–2018.

Evich HB. It feels like something out of a bad sci-fi movie. *Politico,* August 4, 2019.

Intergovernmental Panel on Climate Change. Climate change and land: an IPCC special report. 2019.

Lindsey R. Climate change: atmospheric carbon dioxide. NOAA Climate.gov, February 20, 2020.

Regeneration International. Why regenerative agriculture? 2019.

Scheelbeek PFD, Bird FA, Tuomisto HL, Green R, Harris FB, Joy EJM, et al. Effect of environmental changes on vegetable and legume yields and nutritional quality. *Proceedings of the National Academies of Science, USA.* 2018;115(26):6804–6809.

World Resources Institute. Creating a sustainable food future: a menu of solutions to feed nearly 10 billion people by 2050. Final report, July 2019.

Zhu C, Kobayashi K, Loladze I, Zhu J, Jiang Q, Xu X, et al. Carbon dioxide (CO_2) levels this century will alter the protein, micronutrients, and vitamin content of rice grains with potential health consequences for the poorest rice-dependent countries. *Science Advances.* 2018;4(5):eaaq1012.

16. Will technology fix our food system?

Bollinedi H, Dhakane-Lad J, Krishnan SG, Bhowmick PK, Prabhu KV, Singh NK, et al. Kinetics of β-carotene degradation under different storage conditions in transgenic Golden Rice® lines. *Food Chemistry.* 2019;278:773–779.

Gleizer S, Ben-Nissan R, Bar-On YM, Shamshoum M, Bar-Even A, Milo R. Conversion of Escherichia coli to generate all biomass carbon from CO_2. *Cell.* 2019;179(6):1255–1263.e12.

Nestle M. *Safe Food: The Politics of Food Safety.* Berkeley: University of California Press; 2003. Rev. ed.; 2013.

——. Traditional models of healthy eating: alternatives to techno-food. *Journal of Nutrition Education.* 1994;26:241–245.

——. *What to Eat.* New York: North Point Press / Farrar, Straus and Giroux; 2006.

17. What are Sustainable Development Goals, and why should we care?

Eyal N, Sjöstrand M. On knowingly setting unrealistic goals in public health. *American Journal of Public Health.* 2020;110(4):480–484.

Galatsidas A. Sustainable Development Goals: changing the world in 17 steps—interactive. *The Guardian,* January 19, 2015.

Office of Disease Prevention and Health Promotion. About Healthy People.

Taylor & Francis. Sustainable Development Goals online: a curated library. www.taylorfrancis.com/sdgo/

United Nations. Sustainable Development Goals: knowledge platform. https://sustainabledevelopment.un.org/

United Nations. The Sustainable Development Goals report 2018.

18. Is there a road map to the future of food?

Hirvonen K, Bai Y, Headey D, Masters WA. Affordability of the EAT-Lancet reference diet: a global analysis. *Lancet Global Health.* Published online November 7, 2019.

Swinburn BA, Kraak VI, Allender S, Atkins VJ, Baker PI, Bogard JR, et al. The global syndemic of obesity, undernutrition, and climate change: *The Lancet* Commission report. *Lancet.* 2019;393(10173):791–846.

Willett W, Rockström J, Loken B, Springmann M, Lang T, Vermeulen S, et al. Food in the Anthropocene: the EAT-Lancet Commission on healthy diets from sustainable food systems. *Lancet.* 2019;393(10170):447–492.

Conclusion: Take Action

Association for the Study of Food and Society. This association's website lists food studies programs and resources: www.food-culture.org

Bobo K, Kendall J, Max S. *Organizing for Social Change: Midwest Academy Manual for Activists,* 4th ed. Santa Ana, CA: Forum Press; 2010.

Civil Eats. This site lists food advocacy organizations at https://civileats.com/resources

Food Tank. This group presents "120 organizations creating a new decade for food" at https://foodtank.com/news/2019/12/120-organizations-creating-a-new-decade-for-food

Friends Committee on National Legislation. Advocacy resource: how to meet with Congress. www.fcnl.org/updates/how-to-meet-with-congress-19

Jayaraman S, De Master K, eds. *Bite Back: People Taking On Corporate Food and Winning.* Oakland: University of California Press; 2020. See Hertz J, "Afterword: Taking Action to Create Change," 209–221.

Lee MM, Falbe J, Schillinger D, Basu S, McCulloch CE, Madsen KA. Sugar-sweetened beverage consumption 3 years after the

Berkeley, California, sugar-sweetened beverage tax. *American Journal of Public Health.* 2019;109(4):637–639.

Nestle M. *Soda Politics: Taking on Big Soda (and Winning).* New York: Oxford University Press; 2015.

Pollan M. Big Food strikes back: why did the Obamas fail to take on corporate agriculture? *New York Times,* October 5, 2016.

World Cancer Research Fund. NOURISHING database of implemented policies to promote healthy diets and reduce obesity. www.wcrf.org/int/policy/nourishing-database

Further Reading

Berry W. *Bringing It to the Table: On Farming and Food.* Berkeley, CA: Counterpoint; 2009.

FAO. Nutrition and food systems: a report by the High Level Panel of Experts on Food Security and Nutrition of the Committee on World Food Security. Rome, September 2017.

Gussow JD. *Chicken Little, Tomato Sauce and Agriculture: Who Will Produce Tomorrow's Food?* New York: Bootstrap Press; 1991.

Hauter W. *Foodopoly: The Battle over the Future of Food and Farming in America.* New York: New Press; 2012.

Jayaraman S. *Behind the Kitchen Door.* Ithaca, NY: ILR Press; 2013.

Kuhnlein HV, Erasmus B, Spigelski D. *Indigenous Peoples' Food Systems: The Many Dimensions of Culture, Diversity and Environment for Nutrition and Health.* Rome: FAO and Centre for Indigenous Peoples' Nutrition and Environment; 2009.

Lappé FM. *Diet for a Small Planet,* 20th anniversary ed. New York: Ballantine Books; 1991. 50th anniversary ed.; 2021.

Lerza C, Jacobson M. *Food for People, Not for Profit: A Sourcebook on the Food Crisis.* New York: Ballantine Books; 1975.

Loza M. *Defiant Braceros: How Migrant Workers Fought for Racial, Sexual, and Political Freedom.* Chapel Hill: University of North Carolina Press; 2016.

Miller D. *Farmacology: What Innovative Family Farming Can Teach Us about Health and Healing.* New York: William Morrow; 2013.

Mintz S. *Sweetness and Power: The Place of Sugar in Modern History.* New York: Viking; 1985.

Nesheim MC, Oria M, Yih PT, eds. *A Framework for Assessing Effects of the Food System.* Washington, DC: National Academies Press; 2015.

Patel R. *Stuffed and Starved: The Hidden Battle for the World Food System.* New York: Melville House; 2012.

Penniman L. *Farming While Black: Soul Fire Farm's Practical Guide to Liberation on the Land.* White River Junction, VT: Chelsea Green Publishing; 2018.

Pollan M. *The Omnivore's Dilemma: A Natural History of Four Meals.* New York: Penguin; 2006.

Sbicca J. *Food Justice Now! Deepening the Roots of Social Struggle.* Minneapolis: University of Minnesota Press; 2018.

Schlosser E. *Fast Food Nation: The Dark Side of the All-American Meal.* New York: Houghton Mifflin; 2001.

Simon M. *Appetite for Profit: How the Food Industry Undermines Our Health and How to Fight Back.* New York: Nation Books; 2006.

Wilde P. *Food Policy in the United States: An Introduction.* 2nd ed. Abington, UK: Earthscan; 2020.

Winne M. *Food Rebels, Guerrilla Gardeners, and Smart-Cookin' Mamas: Fighting Back in an Age of Industrial Agriculture.* Boston: Beacon Press; 2010.

INDEX

food-system advocacy
(*continued*)
163–64; to confront climate change, 136–38; to confront overproduction and waste, 99–101; to confront viral health threats, 9; considering an integrated national food policy, 103–4, 108–11; for corporate accountability, 128–30; effective methods for, 166–68; food safety advocacy, 90–91, 94; Global Syndemic report recommendations, 159–60; ideals and goals for, 8–9, 104, 163, 166; to improve the food environment, 77, 165–66; need for, 5–6, 19; SDGs as inspiration for, 152–53; socioeconomic inequities and, 121, 164–65, 166; soda tax advocacy, 165, 167–68; to support regenerative agriculture, 120–21; and technological interventions, 143, 144–45; where to start, 165–66

food systems: defined, 2, 7. *See also* food-system advocacy; sustainable food systems

food waste, 95–101

fortified foods, 48, 53, 54, 58

free-market ideology. *See* food capitalism

fruit juices, 33

fruits and vegetables, 31,32, 33, 41, 59, 123; avoiding pesticides, 93–94; climate change and nutrient content, 134; cost of, 18, 128; school gardens, 83, 85; vegetable proteins, 48, 49, 134.

See also plant-based diets; plant foods; *specific crops*

gardens, in schools, 83, 85

gender disparities, 8, 23, 137, 164

genetically modified (GMO) foods, 93–94, 143–45

global food capitalism, 126–28.

See also food capitalism

global food security, 115–16, 123–24; and climate change, 156; and GMO crops/foods, 143–45; international food aid, 119; the myth of America feeding the world, 115, 116, 118–19, 120; supporting local and regional food security, 119–20; the UN Zero Hunger SDG, 148, 149, 151–52

Global Syndemic report (*The Lancet* commission), 158–60

gluten-free diets. *See* low-carbohydrate diets

glyphosate, 93

GMO foods, 93–94, 143–45

Golden Rice, 144–45

Good Food movement, 163–64

government policies. *See* government regulation; public policy

government regulation and oversight, 5–6, 75; advocating for, 160; and capitalist values, 159; complexity of federal agency authority, 104–7; enforcing existing law, 120; and food safety, 88, 89–91, 94; of the supplement industry, 56–58.

See also food safety; *specific government agencies*

grain-based foods, 32–33

grain-free diets. *See* low-carbohydrate diets

California Studies in Food and Culture

Darra Goldstein, Editor

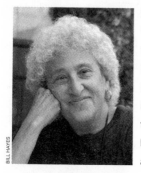

BILL HAYES

Marion Nestle is the Paulette Goddard Professor of Nutrition, Food Studies, and Public Health, Emerita, at New York University, and the author of books about food politics, most recently *Unsavory Truth*. She blogs at www.foodpolitics.com and tweets at @marionnestle.

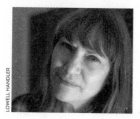

LOWELL HANDLER

Kerry Trueman is an environmental advocate, writer, and consultant who has written about low-impact living, healthy eating, and sustainable agriculture for the *Huffington Post, Civil Eats, AlterNet, and Grist,* among others. She is co-founder of IttyBittyKittyCorner.com, a website offering resources to encourage upcycling, edible landscaping, permaculture, composting, seed saving, and other ecologically sound, technologically savvy ways to cope with the challenges of our ongoing climate and health crises.